A pocket book on
YOGA

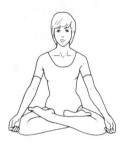

Bob Bury

First published 1982 by
Octopus Books Limited
59 Grosvenor Street
London W1

ISBN 0 7064 1525 6

Produced by Mandarin Publishers Ltd
22a Westlands Road, Quarry Bay, Hong Kong

Illustrations: Coral Mula

Contents

Why do yoga?

There are a variety of reasons for taking up yoga. It can improve health, relieve tension and help you to relax. Some people start because they want to lose weight or make their bodies more supple. This book has been written for the beginner and the lessons in it are designed to take you steadily and without strain through a range of postures. Whatever your reasons for taking up yoga, you are bound to benefit from following this system.

Benefits to the body

If you are ill, the cause is not always the obvious one, as osteopaths have shown time and time again. By adjusting the bone structure, an osteopath can often relieve nervous complaints and blood disorders.

It is basic to yoga that the spine holds the key to an efficient body. Too great a curvature in the dorsal region — rounded shoulders, humped back — prevents the rib-cage expanding properly, which in turn impedes correct breathing, so that the blood is poorly oxygenated, the brain is partially starved and the nervous system is affected. The end result is poor digestion and all that it implies. So, the person with a malformed and rigid spine is vulnerable to illness of one sort or another.

The yogic view is that a body which is fit and supple will have the resistance to ward off illness. Even if you are in good all-round condition, you can use yoga to ensure that you remain so.

Yoga and medicine

But though yoga improves general health, it should be stressed that it can't replace your doctor. If you are ill, you should ask his advice and make sure that your yoga exercises will not conflict with his treatment. Your doctor may even recommend yoga in some cases because it is recognized that if the postures are practised under proper guidance, they can help specific ailments as well as toning up the body generally. But you should check before starting.

The medical profession and those who encourage the practice of yoga often combine in the treatment of psychosomatic illness. The inseparability of body and mind is an acknowledged fact. An overburdened mind disturbs bodily functions, upsets metabolism, raises blood pressure, creates hormone imbalance, and encourages ulcers.

The yoga which tones physique also improves the mind and strengthens character. In fact, the essence of yoga is the development of mind, character and spiritual strength, and the health and beauty so sought after are by-products of a calm mind.

Preparing for yoga

You should never practise yoga until at least two hours after a meal, because the energy required combined with that needed for the digestive process puts undue strain on the stomach. The bladder should be empty too.

Clothing should not restrict movement and must allow the skin to breathe. If you are going to practise in complete privacy, the less clothes you wear the better. For men, a leotard and shorts or gymnastic trousers are ideal. Women should wear a leotard and footless tights; tights do not grip the floor surfaces as well as bare feet. But if you feel the cold you can put on warm socks during relaxation, and cover yourself with a blanket, though it should cover the body without cocooning it. You will need a non-slip mat, and perhaps a small cushion or pad for supporting certain postures and aiding relaxation — the use of such support will be described later.

About the lessons

The instruction in this book is divided into five lessons, graded so that you learn each posture, or asana, in stages. Lesson 1 gives the basic techniques and these should be practised thoroughly before moving on to the next stage. The same postures are then expanded lesson by lesson until the complete processes have been developed so that they are achieved correctly. This method will help you to appreciate the principles of yoga and perform the exercises with concentration and awareness, so that you know them thoroughly and can easily remember every detail. Only seven postures are taught, but these provide a complete programme for practice. Each movement of the body is

5

balanced by a contraposture to prevent strain.

You should allot yourself the same amount of time each day for yoga, and these lessons are based on a 35-minute or a one-hour session, so that you can select the one most suited to your circumstances. The table on page 7 suggests how to break up your session into limbering, relaxation and the postures themselves. Stick to the same length of time — don't do 35 minutes one day and one hour the next.

If you practise for one hour you will include all seven postures each day and you should work on each lesson for a week. If you choose 35 minutes, do only four of the postures each day, varying them so that none is neglected; each lesson should be practised for a fortnight. The book will therefore last you either five or ten weeks, after which you can decide whether to continue with these postures or to find a teacher and learn more — say, at an evening class or yoga club.

What each lesson does

Each lesson has a main theme, contained in the introduction, which should be borne in mind when practising. The first part of each lesson concentrates on relaxation and limbering to prepare the body for the postures. Then there is a pre-limber appropriate for the specific posture before coming to the posture itself. The previous week's development is progressed to the next stage with, wherever possible, points for self-correction. One lesson deals entirely with individual tailoring of the posture to your own shape and physique, so avoiding strain without diminishing the effectiveness of the posture. The contrapostures which follow each posture are designed to balance the muscular effort and relieve tension. The lesson ends with relaxation. Correct breathing is an important part of yoga, and breathing techniques are included in the lessons.

The lessons are designed to be practised in succession. Don't skip any part or try to jump to the last one. Skipping and jumping have no place in yoga and short cuts will not help you.

Now to Lesson 1. Read it through first, studying the pictures and text. In the early stages, though this is not essential, you may like to work with a friend so that one can read the instructions whilst the other carries them out.

YOUR TIMING SYSTEM

1-hour Practice	35-minute Practice
Relax 5 mins,	Relax 3 mins,
Limber 15 mins,	Limber 9 mins,
Postures 25 mins,	Postures 15 mins,
Breathing 7 mins,	Breathing 5 mins,
Relax 8 mins	Relax 3 mins

35 MINUTE PROGRAMME

DAY	PROGRAMME
Monday	*Relax: Limber:* Vrikshasana, Padahastasana, Sarvangasana, Bhujangasana, Breathing, Relaxation.
Tuesday	*Relax: Limber:* Vrikshasana, Janu Shirsasana, Matsyendrasana, Utthita Trikonasana, Breathing, Shavasana.
Wednesday	*Relax: Limber:* Vrikshasana, Viparita Karani or Sarvangasana, Utthita Trikonasana, Bhujangasana, Breathing, Shavasana.
Thursday	*Relax: Limber:* Padahastasana, Bhujangasana, Matsyendrasana, Sarvangasana, Breathing, Shavasana.
Friday	*Relax: Limber:* Padahastasana, Utthita Trikonasana, Matsyendrasana, Janu Shirsasana (with Matsyasana), Breathing, Shavasana.
Saturday	*Relax: Limber:* Vrikshasana, Janu Shirsasana, Sarvangasana, Matsyendrasana, Breathing, Shavasana.
Sunday	*Relax: Limber:* Padahastasana, Utthita Trikonasana, Janu Shirsasana, Bhujangasana, Breathing, Shavasana.

This 35-minute programme can easily be adapted if you wish to practise for one hour. Refer to the timing system given above and remember that seven, rather than four, postures are included in a one-hour session.

LESSON 1

This lesson gives starting points for the five elements which make up each session. These are relaxation, limbering, asana or posture, breathing and quiet concentration. Its theme is 'letting go', observing where tension is, recognizing it and releasing it in relaxation. In each case the benefits of a posture are outlined and there are suggestions for tailoring them to individual characteristics, and any precautions you must take if you have a specific condition, such as back trouble.

Relaxation

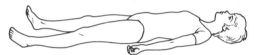

It is a good idea to begin your session with a brief relaxation period. The less tension in mind and body the better they will respond to whatever they have to do. Lie on your back on a mat, arms and legs loosely relaxed. This is the supine (Corpse) position. Lift your head and shoulders and look down at your feet, which should be about 25 cm (10 in) apart. Spread your shoulder blades as wide apart as you can and then gently push your spine down between them and lower your head and shoulders on to the mat. Close your eyes and concentrate on your breathing. Breathe in and feel the coolness. Breathe out steadily. Think about its peaceful regularity. Don't let any other thoughts cross your mind.

Stretching

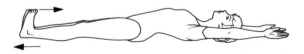

at the same time spread fingers and toes, inhaling fully

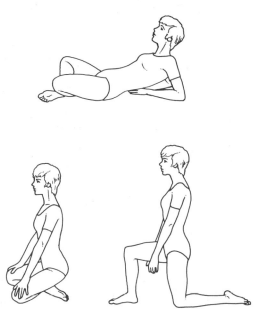

Next, have a good, toning stretch. Take your arms over your head on to the floor, spread your fingers and stretch back, at the same time pulling your well-spread toes towards you and pushing your heels away. Breathe deeply as you do this and, still stretching, breathe out again, bringing the small of your back on to the floor again — it will have lifted off. Relax for a moment. Still lying supine, place both hands under your waist and, breathing in, push yourself up. As you do this, bring your legs up so that you are sitting cross-legged. Continue the forward motion, kneel and then stand. With a little practice you will find you can do this in one easy movement.

Limbering

Limbering prepares the body for the yoga postures by opening up the joints and stretching the muscles, thus avoiding strain from sudden unfamiliar activity. Limbers are an important prelude to the postures.

Forward bend limber

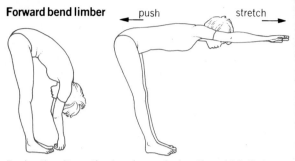

During the alternating tension and relaxation of this limbering exercise, notice which areas in the back, neck, shoulders and legs feel tight.

Stand with the feet about 1 m (3 ft) apart, toes forward, and slowly bend so that the torso hangs loosely. Inhale and bring the upper half of the body parallel with the floor, stretching the arms forward with fingers spread. Push the buttocks back. Breathe slowly out, and lower the trunk to its hanging position with arms and head dangling loosely.

Squat limber

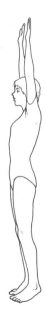

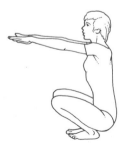

For squats the back must be upright all the time. If you have difficulty with this, work with your back lightly touching a wall or door.

Stand with feet and knees together. Bend into a squat. Stretch your arms in front of you to balance. Try to keep your feet flat, but if you are unable to do this, roll your mat up a little and raise your heels on to the roll. With arms above your head, straighten up as high as you can, coming right on to your toes. Alternate these stretches and squats, breathing in as you rise and out as you descend.

After squats and stretches, kneel back on your heels and relax, noting where the stress areas are.

Flexing limber

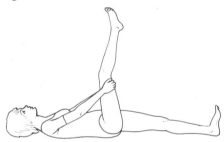

Lie in the supine position, hands by your sides, palms downwards, and raise your left leg about 30 cm (12 ins) from the floor. Flex your left foot backwards and forwards five times, then rotate the toes five times round the ankle joint, first clockwise and then anti-clockwise. Bring the leg straight up, with the toes pointing at the ceiling, and hold the thigh in both hands. Flex the leg at the knee (gently — don't kick with it), then rotate the foot round it both ways, five times in each direction. Repeat with your right leg.

You have limbered ankle and knee joints but there remains the hip. First take your arms out to shoulder level. Bring your left foot against the inside of the right shin, keeping the left knee on the floor. Remember to keep that knee on the floor as the left foot travels up the inside of the right leg to the thigh. Only then will the knee rise up as the leg is re-straightened. This movement can be repeated three times on the left side and three on the right.

Kneeling limber

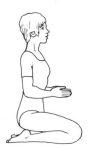
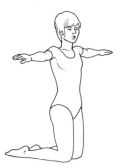

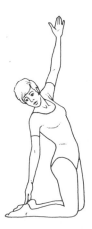

Kneeling on the heels is called Vajrasana in Sanskrit. Kneel with your knees together and feet flattened behind you. Then, with upright but relaxed back and neck, sit back on your heels. Put your hands together as if in prayer but with the fingers pointing forward in the Indian greeting posture (Namasti). Inhaling, rise off your heels to kneel up, and stretch your arms out at shoulder level. Exhaling, take the left arm straight up and, twisting to the right, bring the right hand down to the left heel. Look up to check that the left arm is straight, and then down at the heel you are touching. Sit back on your heels, returning the hands to Namasti. Repeat this with the right arm up.

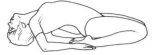

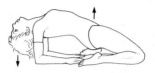

lift right off the heel and allow your head to drop back

Do this three times each way, then part the heels and lean back, supporting yourself either on your hands or on your elbows, depending on how supple you are feeling. Let your head hang loosely back. Inhaling, lift the buttocks high and, exhaling, lower them on to the floor or heels, so arching the lower back. After five or six lifts, lie in the supine position and let tension drain away.

If this limber only gives you a slight feeling of muscular movement, try sinking back on your elbows, again allowing the head to fall back and hang freely, and parting the lips as you do so. There must be no clenching of the jaw. Raise and lower your buttocks.

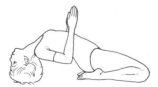

If you are extremely supple you can extend this limber by leaning right back and putting the crown of your head on to the floor. Then bring the hands together (Namasti) on to the abdomen, pointing upwards. This position can be held for five or six breaths before stretching out and relaxing.

13

Scissor limber

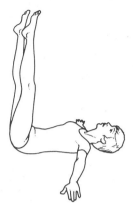

This limber is good for freeing the hip joints. From the supine position, bring both legs upright, spread them out, bring them back together and cross them right over left. Spread them again and cross them left over right. Continue this scissoring motion for a few seconds, quickening it gradually.

Bring your legs down again after doing this limber and relax until you feel ready for your first posture.

The Tree (Vrikshasana)

be sure to keep palms together and elbows back all the time

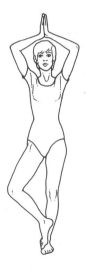

The tree posture involves balancing on one leg, but you should remember that it is a posture and not just a question of balance. To start with, support yourself by touching a wall or a chair lightly with one finger to make sure that the posture is correct. Its purpose is to straighten the legs, but it also stretches the whole body, opens the chest and calms breathing, so achieving body symmetry and correcting any defect in the structure of the spine.

Stand with your feet together, and stretch to your full height. Your weight should rest evenly on the ball of the foot and the heel, and your body be in a straight line from heel to ear. Lengthen upwards without looking upwards. Imagine you are carrying a head-load, so that your upward growth is through the crown of your head. Try not to become rigid and breathe quietly and regularly. Hold this position for a while, then turn your right foot slightly so that the feet are like the hands of a clock at five past twelve. Let your weight fall on the right foot, just steadying your balance with your left big toe. Put your right foot on top of your left one and, breathing in, raise your arms to shoulder level. Bring the palms together, the heels of your hands touching the crown of your head, fingers pointing upward. This hand position is called the Low Mountain. Keep your elbows back, and your body upright and fully lengthened with a straight spine.

Repeat, with the weight on your right foot.

Contraposture: The Child

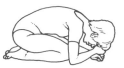

The Child is a simple movement which highlights any tension in the body. Note where you feel tension and try to relax in these places.

Kneel back on your heels and gently lower your head to the floor. Put your arms loosely on to the floor at your sides or, if you find this difficult, make fists, one on top of the other in front of you, as in the illustration, and rest the forehead on them. Relax until you feel no strain at all.

15

The Forward Bend (Padahastasana)

'Pada' means 'foot' and 'hasta' means 'hand', so this is the hand-to-foot posture. It extends the spine, relieving imbalances of pressure on the intervertebral discs. By causing alternating contraction and release round the viscera, whilst conditioning the adrenal glands, it also encourages the flow of gastric juices, stimulates appetite and aids elimination.

But this posture is not advisable for anyone with a 'slipped disc'. Instead you can do more gentle practice on the Cobra, the Fish and the backward bending contraposture for the Forward Bend, which are described on pages 34, 26 and 18.

Limbering

Before attempting the posture itself, practise the two following exercises, to free the back muscles and encourage the flow of sinovial fluid which lubricates the articulating surfaces of the vertebrae.

Stand straight and raise your arms above your head, breathing in. Hold your breath for a moment, then lower your arms to your sides as you breathe out. Spread your feet out to shoulder width and let your arms hang loosely. Your weight should be evenly distributed between the ball of each foot and the heel.

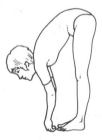 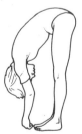

Bring your feet as close together as you comfortably can, keeping them parallel to each other. Then let your whole body hang forward loosely. The abdomen should be relaxed, the arms hanging forward. Shrug your shoulders a few times and let them drop. As you hang forward, look up and then drop your head to relax your neck. Do this several times, so that your head is dangling. You should now be like a rag doll hung over a clothes-line. When you have really relaxed into this position, hold both elbows in the opposite hands. Relax even more. Let the knees give slightly. Breathe rhythmically with a normal intake of air but a long sighing exhalation. Remember that a sigh is a device to relieve tension. Note any point of tightness and try to relax it.

The posture

the arrows indicate where the
alternations of stretch and
release take place

You are now ready for the Forward Bend. Stand with your feet close together, then stretch upwards breathing in fully. As you exhale, bend your knees, keeping them close together, until you can grip your toes. Breathe in, look up and hollow your back as much as you can. Breathe out again, meanwhile bending your face towards your knees. Still gripping the toes, straighten your legs as much as you comfortably can, rounding your back. Repeat these two movements several times until the whole spine feels loosely pliant.

This preparatory posture is sometimes called padangusta-sana because padangusta means the big toe round which you can loop your fingers. When in the first position, knees bent and head up, think about also lifting the back of your pelvis towards the ceiling. In the second position do not strain to put your head on your knees, but think in terms of dropping your head, crown first, on top of your feet.

17

Contraposture

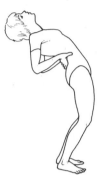

After bending the spine in a forward direction, you must bend it backwards to compensate.

Stand with feet about 25-30 cm (10-12 ins) apart, with the toes pointing forwards. Put both hands on your hips, with the thumbs pointing forwards and fingers down. The heels of the hands should press into the waist. Breathe in deeply and, as you slowly breathe out, increase the pressure of your hands and let your entire spine, including the vertebrae of the neck, arch backward. Part the lips to avoid tension in the neck. Keep your feet flat on the floor and let your knees give slightly to balance. If you find this difficult, you can raise your heels a bit, on a pad or rolled-up mat.

Relaxation

Lie supine on the floor, the limbs spread symmetrically. Concentrate on any area where you felt stress. Be conscious of this area each time you breathe out. If the small of your back tends to arch away from the floor, draw your feet close against your buttocks, the knees together and pointing upward.

This posture is found to be more relaxing if the feet are kept flat on the floor, some 18 inches apart. Each person being differently structured, the test here is whether or not you yourself actually feel relaxed. Whether you have your knees touching or not, your arms close to your body or not, your palms facing up or down, are things for you to decide.

The Stretched Triangle
(Utthita Trikonasana)

This posture, as the name suggests, stretches the body into
a triangle. It actually creates two triangles, one being made
by the floor between the feet and the straight legs, and the
other being formed by the side of the trunk, an arm and a
leg. It gives a strong stretch to the hip joint, lengthening the
associated muscles.

In the Stretched Triangle, the muscles of the legs are
firmed, the spine is kept supple, the chest is opened and
that area of the flank where fat accumulates is massaged.

Limbering

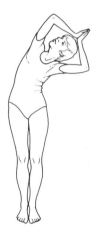

Stand straight, as you did before starting the Tree posture.
Lengthen, but comfortably, 'through the crown'. Breathe
in steadily and put your hands into the Low Mountain
position. Do not let the elbows come forward. As you
breathe out, look at the right elbow and bend to the left as
far as you can. Keep the movement sideways — don't move
forwards. Straighten up, breathing in. Bend to the right as
you breathe out, looking at your left elbow. Repeat these
limbering bends at least three times on each side; then
stand straight but relaxed, breathing evenly.

The posture

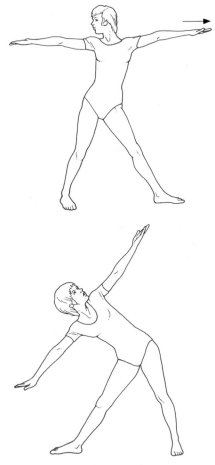

Stand with feet astride at a comfortable distance apart. To find the best astride position for you, stand with your feet together and see how long a stride forward you can take without lifting the heel of the rear foot from the floor. This distance is the right one for you. Point the left foot sideways, keeping the trunk still. Do this in two movements — first pivot on the heel some 45° and then on the ball of the foot, swinging the heel to point towards the middle of the right foot.

Whilst doing this you should be keeping the torso and pelvis quite still. Avoid body-turn. If you do this correctly you will feel exactly where your hip-joint is, which is important. Do not confuse hips with the area of the waist. As you become more aware of the hip joint you will be able to feel its movement with your fingers as you point the foot. Experiment. Feel the motions of this joint as you move your knees and ankles in other ways: for instance, in the flexing limber described on page 11. You will become aware of its great importance and the need to maintain it in free working order.

Now with the feet correctly positioned, breathe in, raising the arms to shoulder level and then look at them. Make sure they are quite level. As you breathe in again, turn your head to look along your right arm. Breathing out, bend slowly as far to the left as you can without straining. Try to maintain the 'T' shape, and with an in-breath stand upright again. Repeat the posture pointing the right foot outward and bending to the right.

Make sure that you avoid any forward movement of the body during this posture. Imagine that you are in a narrow box. This will limit your sideways movement. It is far better to manage a limited version honestly than to perform a great bend incorrectly.

Take care, too, that your arms stay in the 'T' pattern. Try doing this posture close to a wall. First face the wall, then stand with your back to it, the hand bent slightly back at the wrist so that the finger-tips can maintain contact with the wall throughout the posture. When you reach your limit each time, pause in that position for three or four quiet breaths.

While you pause, concentrate on knees, legs, back, neck and shoulders, noting any ache or rigidity. Consciously relax where you feel any tightness. Try to double the length of your breathing out. If you cannot do this you are straining and must come out of the posture.

The contraposture

This posture compensates for the effort put into not leaning forward in the Stretched Triangle. Stand with the legs in the

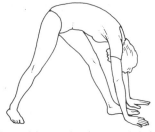

same astride position and point your left foot to the left. Take a full breath and raise the arms straight up, at the same time turning the trunk to the left. Let your breath out gradually and bring the trunk down, your hands touching the floor to balance. You may have to bend the forward knee very slightly to put your hands on the floor. The top of your head should be in line with your left foot. Take three or four quiet, relaxing breaths, then stand up as you breathe in. Do this again in the opposite direction.

Relaxation

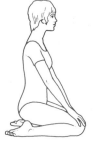

It only takes a few seconds for muscle fibres to regain their shape after being stretched, but it is important to relax after a posture to enable them to do this. A pleasant posture in which to release tension is Vajrasana, described on page 12. An alternative is to part the heels and sit between them, a position known as Gorakshasana.

The Single Leg Forward Stretch
(Janu Shirsasana)

Janu Shirsasana translates as 'face to knee'. This means that the face is pointed towards the knee, not necessarily that the two should touch.

The main effects of this posture are to stretch the muscles of each leg in turn, to ease the hip joint, to correct and lengthen the spine and to encourage a flow of fresh blood to the spleen, pancreas and kidneys. Digestion and elimination are thus assisted by this posture and it should also be practised regularly by anyone suffering from an enlarged prostate gland. But you must be careful if you have a painful back and you shouldn't do it at all if you have slipped a disc. You can substitute the Fish posture (Matsyasana), which is also the contraposture for this section (see page 26).

Limbering

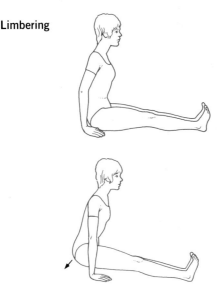

allow the seating bones to move back

This exercise loosens the hip joints, making the posture itself easier to manage. Sit on the floor with your legs straight out in front of you, and your hands on the floor, pointing forwards. Keeping your legs straight, lift your buttocks off the floor, leaning forward at the same time. Sit on the mat again and straighten your body. You can do this several times.

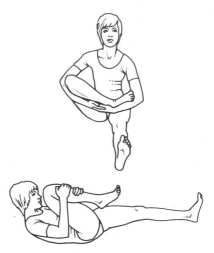

The following limbering exercise loosens the hip joints too. Sit with your legs out in front of you as you did for the last limber. Pick up your left foot and lodge it firmly in the crook of your right elbow. Pass your left forearm under the lifted knee and join your hands. Now 'rock the baby' as freely as you can, from side to side and up and down. Then lie back as shown in the picture above, clasp your shin with both hands and try to make head and knee touch.

The posture

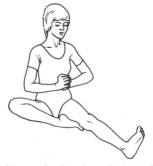

Sit in the same position as for the above limbers. Draw the left foot up so that its sole lies along the inside of the right thigh. Do not allow the foot to burrow its way under the thigh. If your knee will not rest on the floor despite the limbering exercises, don't force it. Practice will help you to achieve this in time. When you have got as far as you can into the posture, try to stay in that position for 10 or 20 seconds.

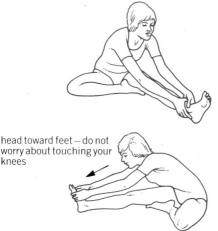

head toward feet – do not worry about touching your knees

Bend from the hips, not the waist, as you breathe out slowly. Try to put your abdomen on the thigh of your straight leg. Grip the leg round the ankle or, if you can't reach this far, as low down the leg as is comfortable. You can bend your knee slightly if you have difficulty, gently trying to straighten it as you bend further forward. Keep your eyes on your toes and, as you slowly exhale, bend the elbows downward towards your mat, drawing the whole trunk down. Hold your foot if you can.

Try to keep your back straight during this posture. Do not round your shoulders trying to reach your knee with your head. Push the crown of your head towards your foot. Think of lengthening as you breathe in, and relaxing downwards as you breathe out.

When you come out of the posture, keep the spine straight and bend from the hips into the start position, stretching your arms straight above your head as you breathe in. Breathing out, put your arms by your sides again and straighten the bent leg. Repeat the posture, drawing up the right foot and stretching along the left leg.

Contraposture: The Fish (Matsyasana)

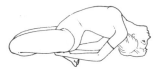

You are bound to feel some tightness during the Single Leg Forward Stretch. An effective posture to balance this is the Fish, which is also the posture to substitute for the Single Leg Forward Stretch if you have a slipped disc.

Lie supine, arms by your sides, palms down and legs crossed. Supporting yourself on your elbows, grip the feet, arch your spine and drop your head back to rest the crown on the floor. Keep your buttocks on the floor. Flatten the abdominal region as much as possible and concentrate on using rib movement in your breathing. Hold the posture for a few seconds, then lie supine again.

Relaxation

The Raised Corpse posture (Shavasana) with knees brought together and raised is ideal for loosening thighs and hamstrings after the last exercise. Lie on your back with arms out by your sides, and feet apart. Draw your feet up along the floor until they are close to the buttocks. This posture also relaxes the back and hips.

Sitting Rotation (Matsyendrasana)

Matsyendra was a sage of ancient India and this posture is named after him. It rotates the abdominal and thoracic regions around the spine, releasing the spinal muscles and freeing lesions of the spine itself. Resulting benefits are a healthy blood supply to the kidneys and liver and efficient working of the adrenal glands. Sitting Rotation, and the twisting postures leading up to it, relieve backache and stiffness in neck and shoulders. The posture also massages the intestines, preventing constipation.

Anyone suffering from stomach pains should take this gently, and people with hiatus hernia should not do it all.

Limbering

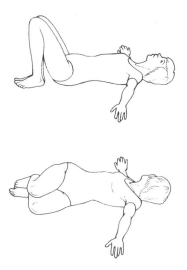

You can go into your limbering routine straight from the Corpse position used for relaxation after the last posture. Lie supine with knees raised, and, keeping the knees pointing upwards, bring the feet together on the floor as close to the buttocks as possible. With palms turned down, bring your arms out sideways at shoulder level.

Breathe in, turning your head to the left. Breathe out, bringing your knees down onto the floor on your right. Try to keep your knees touching each other all the way over. Do not let your toes leave the floor if you can help it, and keep your arms and shoulders flat against the floor. Breathe in, bringing the knees up again and turn your head over to the right. Breathe out, bringing the knees down on the left.

Notice that the head and knees go in opposite directions and that the knees are always lowered as you breathe out. Repeat this 'knee roll' three more times on each side, then stretch the legs and relax.

Put your hands under the small of your back and push up into a sitting position, legs out in front of you.

The posture

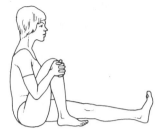

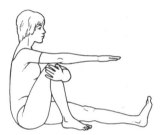

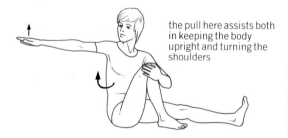

the pull here assists both
in keeping the body
upright and turning the
shoulders

Sit on the floor with legs outstretched in front of you. Bring
up your left knee so that the foot is alongside your right
thigh. Hug this knee, putting both hands round it, and
lengthen your whole body up out of the pelvis. Keep a
straight spine throughout this posture.

Extend the left arm forward, looking along it. Keep the eyes
riveted on that hand and, as you breathe slowly out, circle it
to the left until it is pointing — and you are looking —
backwards. Anyone looking down on you should see a leg,

28

your head and an arm all in a straight line. Your shoulders should have turned through 90 degrees. Hold this position for as long as you comfortably can. Then breathe in and circle the hand forward again. Release and straighten the knee, taking the hands down on to the thighs. Draw up the right knee, hugging it and lengthening up again, ready to repeat the posture to the right. In this case, the rotation in one direction is itself a contraposture to the opposite rotation.

Relaxation

Rest in the forward sitting position for a short while and then repeat this twist of the spine once to the left and once more to the right. As you do this the second time note where your tensed-up areas are. Are you tight in the neck, the shoulders, under the shoulders, in the lumbar area of the spine? Has the straight leg gone rigid? Be really aware of these stress points and, without losing your upright posture, try to relax them. Let go.

A good relaxation exercise after spinal rotations is the Swimmer.

heels turned slightly outward

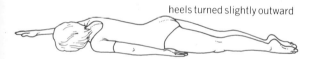

Lie on your front with your feet slightly apart, heels turned a little outward. Let the left arm lie loosely at your side, palm upward, and the right arm stretch ahead of you, palm down. Turn your head to the right, your face towards your right arm so that you are effectively breathing through one nostril. Every ten breaths or so, reverse the arm positions and turn your head to the other side.

The Shoulder Stand (Sarvangasana)

As the English name suggests, this is an inverted posture. The word 'sarva' in the Sanskrit name means 'all', and this exercise is beneficial to the whole body. It improves the blood supply to the thyroid and parathyroid glands which play an important role in growth and metabolism. It makes the scalp and facial tissues firm, helps relieve varicose veins, and is an excellent posture for all-round toning of the body. It draws any mucus out of lungs and into the bronchial area, from where it can be coughed away, eases the digestive processes, and has a calming effect on the nervous system generally. And, because so many supporting and balancing muscles are at work, the posture causes a drain-back of fats from their storage areas in the liver and abdominal wall, thus diminishing weight and obesity without overworking the heart.

WARNING As so much muscular activity is involved, anyone with cardiac weaknesses or high blood pressure should not do the shoulder stand for any length of time. It is better not to do it at all during menstrual periods because the blood released at this time is often very acid and a back-flow could damage the womb. Others who should avoid inversions generally are those who suffer ear discharge or displaced retina. Instead, double your session on the Forward Bend or the Single Leg Forward Stretch, interspersing them with plenty of relaxation.

Like all the postures described in this book, the full Shoulder Stand will not be achieved until later, and in this lesson we will start with the Half Candle posture.

Limbering

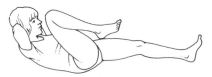

do not strain — as close as you can get is close enough

Lie supine, your hands joined behind your head. As you breathe in, press down on your elbows and raise your chest. Breathe out, letting your back sink on to the floor again, and pull your head forward to look at your feet. Repeat this five or six times to loosen the neck and shoulders. Relax for a few seconds. Breathing in, draw one leg against the chest. Breathing out, lift head and shoulders off the mat and try to touch forehead to knee, which will lengthen the dorsal and cervical sections of your spine. Repeat this with the other leg.

Another useful limber is to raise one leg straight up, with your hands supporting it just above the knee, and flex the knee gently. Repeat this with the other leg, and then with both legs.

The Half Candle

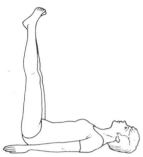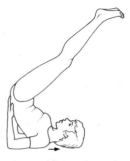

lengthen and flatten the neck

The Half Candle is sometimes known as Viparita Karani, meaning in Sanskrit 'performing in reverse'. In this posture the back forms an angle with the floor. It is not upright, like the complete Shoulder Stand; the legs should be at right angles to the trunk.

Lie on your back, raise your knees and straighten both legs into a vertical position so that your body and legs are in an L-shape. Anyone who has variocose veins or tired feet can practise this part of the posture on its own several times a day to ease them. It is very restful if you use a wall to support your legs.

Continue the movement upwards so that your feet go above your head and your back lifts off the floor. Support it at the waist with both hands.

If you have difficulty in raising your back off the floor, practise against a wall as suggested for the L-posture. Help yourself up by pressing your feet against the wall, bringing them above your head only when you are supporting your back with your hands. When you are comfortable, put your hands flat on the floor. Observe that your diaphragm is now operating differently from when you are upright so think about the part it is playing in the process of breathing. Check that your chin is not locked against your chest, and try to lengthen your neck slightly. There are seven smaller

31

vertebrae in the neck and some people have a more prominent seventh one at the root of the neck. This can cause
discomfort in shoulder standing postures and those who
experience this are advised to place a small pad or cushion
high between the shoulder blades so as to relieve this
pressure.

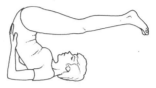

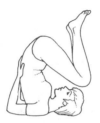

As you come out of the Half Candle your head should not
rise from the floor. To make sure of this, first bring the feet
down so that you are looking up at your knees. With your
legs as close to your face as possible, gently lower your back
on to the floor, bringing your legs into the vertical position.
Try to feel your vertebrae touching down one by one. If you
find it difficult to do this at first, bend your legs as in the
picture, rather than straining the stomach muscles.

Contraposture
There may have been a tightness in the dorsal and abdominal sinews during the last posture. To reverse these
stretches, do the Fish posture described on page 26, but
stretch your arms above your head to release tension in
elbows and wrists.

Relaxation
After all this lifting of the back and legs, it is best to relax in
the supine position, feet slightly apart and dropped loosely

outwards, back well supported on the floor, arms evenly angled out from the torso and shoulder blades well parted. Use this posture, too, to regain balanced breathing, mentally counting the in and out breaths, and making sure that they are regular after the emphasis that has been placed on the abdominal aspect of breathing.

The Cobra (Bhujangasana)

The Sanskrit word 'Bhujanga' actually means 'serpent', not 'cobra'. The posture is called the Cobra because it looks rather like a cobra's hood spreading as the creature rises from the ground.

Think how often you arch your spine forward: crouching over the wheel of a car, attending to the children, putting coal on the fire or even tying a shoe lace. But the spine is rarely curved backwards. This is why some people develop a stoop. The Cobra, which bends the spine backward, corrects deteriorating posture. It also tones the adrenal, thyroid and parathyroid glands, is good for the kidneys, stretches the muscles of the abdomen, and opens the chest.

If you have a slipped disc which is not too well established, the Cobra posture, performed with care, can help, but do not attempt this without your doctor's advice.

Limbering

rise on out breath

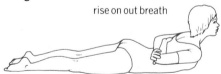

Turn into the prone (face downward) position with your arms by the side of your body, palms to the floor. Concentrate on those long, powerful sinews which stretch from your waist right up under your shoulder blades. Try to control them. Flex them, alternately tightening and releasing. You will find that they operate in conjunction with the strong muscles which draw in the abdomen. Fold your arms behind you, over the small of your back, and breathe in deeply. Then, breathing out slowly, raise your head and

33

chest off the floor, using only those same muscles. Lower again as soon as you have reached your limit. Do not strain. Rest.

The posture

Everyone can do this posture but do not expect everyone to look the same. Some people are naturally more pliant than others. Work to your own limits. Never mind how far someone else bends; it is *your* back we are interested in. When performing this posture, concentrate on two factors. Firstly, the lower abdomen, or the front of the pelvic bone, must be kept in contact with the floor. Secondly, the shoulders must not be hunched: keep them down even if this means bending the elbows slightly.

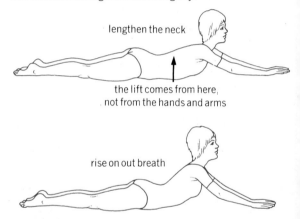

lengthen the neck

the lift comes from here,
not from the hands and arms

rise on out breath

Lie prone and stretch your arms out in front of you, as though you had just dived into some water. As you breathe in, lengthen your neck, pushing your head forward and up. Then, breathing out, pull the chest and torso even further up, pressing the palms down to support. Now relax into the prone position again, the arms still outstretched. Bring the fingernails of your right hand level with your left wrist, then draw your left hand level with the right one. You have drawn your hands in towards your head by one hand's length. Repeat the movement, raising the back higher.

Try to keep the breath under steady control, using a quick, full intake and slow, sighing exhalation. Centre the mind on the muscles in the back and abdomen, consciously relaxing them throughout the seven or eight breaths during which you will hold the posture.

Contraposture
The Child posture (see page 15) compensates for the back stretching of the Cobra.

Relaxation
Relax into the Swimmer posture described on page 29. This will quickly ease the tightened muscles of the back into a pleasant state of freshly-toned rest.

Breathing

Correct breathing is an important part of yoga because it is an important part of relaxation and calm.

Breathing is of course the means by which the body systems are fuelled. Without oxygen neither mind nor muscles will function. But it also affects the nervous system and is a way of controlling emotion and restoring calm. The old remedy of counting ten if you are angry or disturbed can be applied to breathing. Count ten full deep breaths and you will feel calmer.

Here then are a few preliminary exercises for developing correct breathing.

Exercises
Sit cross-legged, or in the upright kneeling posture, sitting back on your heels (Vajrasana). Or you can sit on a chair with your feet together on the floor in front of you and your back completely straight against the chair back. It is important to keep the whole spine perfectly straight. Keep the lower jawline parallel to the floor and allow your arms to fall loosely forward, the backs of your hands resting on your knees.

Now breathe, keeping your mind on the breathing. Use the whole thorax. Let the abdomen go slack as you begin each breath, then raise the rib cage to expand the lungs, flattening the abdomen. As you breathe out again, release the abdomen, then the rib-cage, again flattening the abdomen. Try to practise this rhythmically for two or three minutes then test the pace of your pulse. Count the beats to the minute. Now at the same speed, breathe in for a four-count, then out for a four-count, and pause for two. Continue this breath-pattern of 4-4-2, 4-4-2, for a little while. Later you may be able to extend this, according to your lung capacity, to 6-6-3 or even 8-8-4. But don't strain and if you have any heart weakness don't hold your breath; just breathe 4-4 or 6-6 or 8-8.

Relaxation

Lie in the supine position. Make sure that your whole body is symmetrical: imagine a straight line through your nose and over your navel extending to the level of your feet. The arms and legs should be at equal angles from that line. The angle does not matter so long as the limbs are symmetrical. Have the arms loose but straight, the palms turned upward. Alternately clench and extend the fingers and toes, finally letting the feet drop outward from each other.

Now tighten and relax all the way along the body from the feet to the scalp. Brace your knee-caps and let go until they feel relaxed. Treat thigh and buttock muscles the same way and also pull in and release the solar plexus.

Clench your fists and bend them up, keeping your wrists on the floor, and so harden the arm and shoulder muscles right up to your ears.

Draw in the chin and lengthen the neck, screw up all your facial muscles, frown and tighten the scalp.

Then let everything relax with a long sigh. Let your index fingers lightly touch against your thumbs and allow your upper teeth to rest lightly on your lower lip.

Breathe through the nose. Your respiration should now be light and rather slower. It should also be almost entirely by the diaphragm. Expand the abdomen gently upward and outward as you inhale and let it contract as you exhale.

Keep your mind on this motion of the breath for a little while, then let your mind wander to some pleasant thought. After a pause, return to conscious breathing with a gradual increase of breath, taking it into the upper lungs and peacefully stretching your whole body, bringing your arms overhead, pushing your heels away, pulling your toes towards you, and flattening your back against the floor.

Finally, relax again briefly as you sigh out.

LESSON 2

Relaxation, limbering, basic breathing, and the initial forms of the seven postures will by now have given you a greater awareness of your body, its muscular sensations and its individual limitations. You should also have learnt your own limits, so avoiding strain, but you should still be careful not to overdo it.

The symptoms of strain are trembling; shortness of breath; heavy perspiration; over-rapid pulse-beat in the throat, head or chest; dizziness; and, of course, pain. If you feel any of these, relax at once.

The theme of this lesson is lengthening. Each stage will concentrate on correcting excess spinal curvature and separating the vertebrae, leading to greater suppleness and improvement in carriage. The limbering and contra-posture, unless otherwise specified, is the same as for each posture in Lesson 1, and this applies throughout the book.

Relaxation

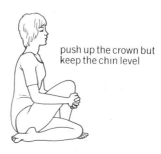

push up the crown but keep the chin level

Begin with relaxation in the Quarter Lotus Posture. Sit with your legs in front of you. Pass the left foot under the right knee, bringing it up against the right buttock. Draw the right foot in towards you and take it across to the outside of the left knee. The right knee will be raised in front of you. Clasp both hands round it, bringing the spine up out of the pelvis straight and tall.

Close your eyes, breathe evenly and quietly, relaxing and allowing your weight to sink down into the pelvic basin. Remember that relaxing and collapsing are two entirely different things. Let your back remain effortlessly straight. Depending on the routine you have selected, relax in this

37

posture for three or five minutes. Then give yourself a long steady stretch, supine on the floor, and relax again into the Corpse Posture.

The Tree (Vrikshasana)

Limbering

Lie supine and take your arms back behind your head. Try to touch the floor with your shoulder, elbow, wrist and finger nails. Hold this position for a few breaths. Straighten the arms as much as you can. Stand up and stretch your arms into exactly the same position as you breathe in, bringing them slowly to your sides as you breathe out. Do this twice more and incorporate it with the limbering exercises you learned in Lesson 1.

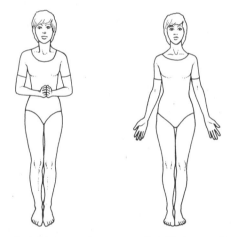

Another limbering exercise you can do is Tadasana. Stand with feet together and hands by your sides. Breathe out and bring your hands together over your stomach, fingers pointing forward in the Namasti position. Breathe in, turning the hands out at your sides, palms forward and thumbs back. As you do this 'grip the floor' with your toes, brace the knees, firm the buttocks and draw in the abdomen. Drop the shoulders and lengthen the neck, without tilting up the chin. Relax and return hands over your stomach. Repeat four times.

The posture

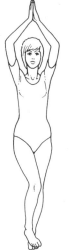

As the theme of this lesson is lengthening, the spine is stretched more than in Lesson 1 by having the hands in the High Mountain position instead of the Low Mountain.
Stand with the right foot covering the left as in Lesson 1. Breathe in and take the arms into the High Mountain position, palms flat together and stretched to maximum height. Breathe out, coming slowly down. Repeat on the other leg. Do each side twice.

The Forward Bend (Padahastasana)

In Lesson 1, you gripped the feet with knees bent. This time the body is stretched further by keeping the legs straight during the posture.

Limbering

Limber and practise the first stage of the posture as in Lesson 1. Breathe in and raise your arms really straight above your head. As you exhale, swing your hands forward and down, bending the knees slightly, until the toes can be gripped. Alternate flattening and rounding of the back, knees bending and stretching, with the breathing as in Lesson 1. Finish by hanging loosely forward, as before. Now stretch up hard with the thumbs linked together.

The posture

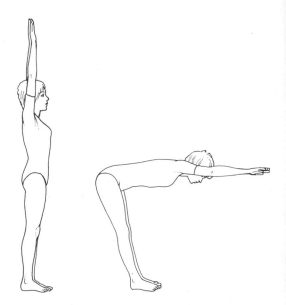

Stand upright, arms above your head and touching your ears. Draw yourself up to your full height as you breathe in. Breathing out, slowly bring the trunk parallel with the floor. Breathe in, hollow your back, push the hips backward and the hands forward, lengthening from buttocks to finger nails. Then, breathing out gently, allow your whole body to relax loosely downward. Keeping the legs straight, grip the toes with both hands, or failing this, join the fingers behind the lower legs.

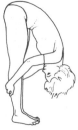

The Stretched Triangle
(Utthita Trikonasana)

In this exercise too, you will continue the stretching process, bending further into the triangle than before.

Limbering
Limber as you did in Lesson 1, but as an additional limber stand with your feet comfortably astride and practise pushing your hip to one side while keeping your arms and torso in a T-shape. Keep the right shoulder vertically above the left as you push your torso right over from the hips. Repeat the posture to the right. Take an equal number of breaths on each side.

The posture

this arm, remaining parallel to the floor, reaches strongly sideways

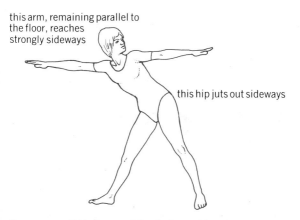

this hip juts out sideways

Start as you did in Lesson 1 but before taking the trunk over to the left, push the right hip outward. Look along the right arm and stretch the left one sideways as far as you can, keeping the arms parallel to the floor.

You can use the wall to practise this. Stand with the feet correctly placed and arms at shoulder level. Look away from the wall and reach sideways until you can touch it. Do not let the trunk sway forward. Try it a little further from the wall until you have reached your limit. Of course you must practise reaching in both directions equally.

41

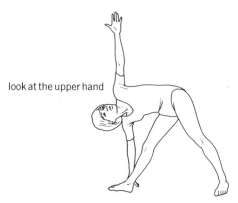

look at the upper hand

Breathe in deeply then, as you slowly breathe out, lean the trunk to the left. This movement should be sideways only with no forward bending in it. Watch the right hand as it stretches vertically into the air. Each time you breathe out, bend a little further, making sure the trunk does not incline forwards, until you can touch the floor with your left hand. Repeat the posture bending to the right, for an equal number of breaths.

The Single Leg Forward Stretch
(Janu Shirsasana)

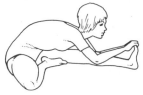

Repeat the limbering and first stages of the posture from Lesson 1, then proceed to the next stage. Sitting with your legs outstretched in front of you, draw up the foot, bending out the knee as in Lesson 1, then raise the arms so that, with the thumbs linked, the upper arms touch the ears. Stretch up. Now, leading with the abdomen again, hinge the trunk forward from the hips so that you can grip the feet. The leg should be kept straight and the elbows bent down as far as possible to stretch the back. But don't strain. The stretching required here is done as you breathe in. As you breathe out release all abdominal tightness and let your body relax easily down on to your leg. Try not to round your back. You must lengthen right along your back and neck, and also along your leg from heel to buttock. To do this more easily it is helpful to rock a little from side to side.

Retain this posture for the same number of breaths on each side, but guard against strain. You may well find that you function more efficiently on one side than on the other. If this is the case, make a note of your worse side and always practise that first whilst your muscular energy is at its highest level.

Sitting Rotation (Matsyendrasana)

In Lesson 1, the first stage of this posture, with the knee raised, practised rotating the trunk round the spine whilst ensuring that it remained erect. The movement in this lesson introduces an element of stretch against the hip joint. There is also a considerable easing of the shoulder joint, which must be supple for the final posture.

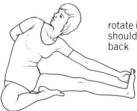

rotate in order at waist, shoulders and neck — look back

Assume the same sitting position as at the start of the Single Leg Forward Stretch, with the left leg stretched forward and the right knee bent outward on the floor, the foot high on the inner side of the left thigh. Keep the back as erect as you can and with the left hand reach to grip the toes of the left foot. Retaining this grasp and breathing in, stretch the right hand out at shoulder level and lengthen the body tall and straight. As you breathe out, look along the outstretched arm and turn it to point behind you, then, on reaching your maximum rotation to the right, bend the elbow, pushing the arm behind your back. Push round

43

further on your next breath out, trying to put your fingers on the straight left thigh. Reverse the posture.

The shoulders will rotate through a good 90 degrees in each direction, and it is important that the posture should, if possible, be sustained for an equal number of breaths on each side.

The Shoulder Stand (Sarvangasana)

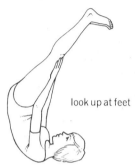

look up at feet

The two postures in this lesson progress further towards the Shoulder Stand, though they are postures in their own right. The first is the Pose of Tranquillity (Viparita Karani), so called because it is very restful. It begins like the posture in Lesson 1 but, when you feel well balanced, you put your hands on to your thighs. A common error is to let your feet go back too far, so that you are looking up at your knees instead of your feet.

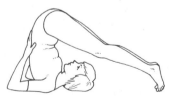

The second posture is called the Plough (Halasana). 'Hala' means a plough and the shape of the posture does resemble a plough. It is an excellent posture for relieving stiffness in the shoulders and neck, massaging the abdominal organs and toning the thyroid glands. From the Pose of Tranquillity, lengthen the neck, support your back again and, keeping your legs straight, bring them right over your head to touch the floor with your toes if you can. Stay in this position for a while, breathing regularly. If you find your breathing is restricted don't overdo it at this stage — just concentrate on trying to get as far into the posture as you can. You will learn more about holding the posture and breathing easily in Lesson 3.

The Cobra with dynamics
(Bhujangasana)

The dynamic in this lesson intensifies the whole Cobra posture learnt in Lesson 1. The leg movement tenses the buttocks and anus, and tightens the abdominal muscles which in turn pull against sinews in the thorax. But it is a very vigorous version of the Cobra so do not overdo it.

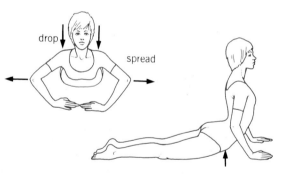

contact with floor

Begin by practising the stages of the Cobra learnt in Lesson 1, taking hands back until finger tips meet under forehead thus increasing the extent of back lift. Hold the final stage — hands on the floor under the shoulders, head well back, and spine arched back as much as you comfortably can — for several breaths. If your shoulders have hunched, bend your elbows out to drop them, without releasing the posture forward. As you breathe in each time, relax your back and let more of the abdominal region touch the floor.

45

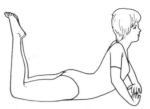

Now as you breathe out, bend the knees so that your feet are pointing straight up in the air. Because this causes the buttocks, abdomen, and chest to feel tense, you shouldn't try to hold the posture.

Concentrate on your breathing during this exercise as it will feel more restricted than usual. Focus your attention on the rib-cage, making it rise and fall as you breathe.

The Snake Dynamic

This dynamic of the Cobra adds a rotational element to the posture. One effect of it is to squeeze the liver, stimulating a healthy blood-flow to that important cleansing organ. The spine itself is activated, stimulating the fluid production between its sinovial surfaces and correcting any inclination to slipped discs between the vertebrae. Like all twisting movements, it creates a massaging effect on the viscera and the colon, helping the bowels to work more efficiently. Again, there will be some restriction in breathing and you should look out for any sign of strain.

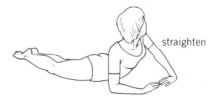

straighten

Work through the stages of the Cobra until you reach the full posture, but with the fingertips of each hand pointing towards each other. The shoulders should not be raised, but stretching should be in the lengthening of the neck with head back. Correct your posture as necessary and hold it long enough to acquire a gentle, steady pattern of breath. Straighten your left arm and bend the right one so that the

46

forearm lies on the floor. Breathing out, turn your head to the left to look over your shoulder at your heels. Breathing in, resume the normal posture. Breathing out, straighten your right arm, bend the left one and look over the right shoulder. Keep the neck long. Repeat the dynamic once or twice.

To build up heavy tension is not the objective of any yoga posture. The very supple person will do these two dynamics with ease, much benefit and probably some pride. The less supple person may become short of breath, trembling and perspiring and should stop to relax thoroughly. You should also pride yourself on recognising your own limitations.

Breathing

In Lesson 1, the breathing exercise was 'triangular' — that is, there were three stages. Here it is 'square' because an extra stage has been added.

Before you start, check that you are counting in time with your pulse beat. Sit symmetrically and erect, looking straight ahead. Breathe in steadily for a count of four, hold your breath for another four, breathe out evenly for a further count of four, and wait for four, before starting the next round. This completes the square. Breathe six squares.

	Retain for 4	
Inhale for 4		Exhale for 4
Start	WAIT for 4	

Your heart and lungs work in very close harmony, the heart pumping venous blood to the lungs where it is cleansed and re-oxygenated. The lungs return it to the heart, as arterial blood, for circulation to the tissues. Naturally the two brain centres which govern these good partners are closely situated and in intimate neural communication. We know that if we stimulate the action of the lungs by exaggerated heavy breathing we increase the heart's activity and raise our blood pressure. By the same token, if we are able to gain control of our breathing rate and steady it we can also slow down the heart's rhythm of pulsation. For this reason, in seeking to relax body or mind — or, indeed, both for they are inseparable — it makes obvious sense to steady the respiration. We do this unconsciously in normal sleep, thus lowering the pulse-rate, resting the heart and decreasing the intake and distribution of unrequired oxygen.

Square breathing is a very good introduction to control of breath and according to your natural lung capacity you can progress from a 4-4-4-4 ratio to a 6-6-6-6 ratio or even 8-8-8-8 and then carry this rhythmic practice forward into your relaxation.

Relaxation

The Corpse posture described in Lesson 1 is used again but to it is added an imagination exercise. First assume the Corpse position, letting your body sink into the floor, a dead weight.

Two main regions of the body are most vulnerable to tension. One is the abdomen, where those 'butterflies' live. Ease tension by 'breathing with the diaphragm'; let the abdominal region extend and decrease with your breath, softly and regularly. The other area, where we bridle when indignant, is the nape of the neck. If you feel at all uneasy there, raise your head slightly on a small pad, a cushion, or two or three books. And don't feel guilty about lying there doing nothing. You have a *right* to relax. It is good for you. *Enjoy it.*

Now, as you breathe in the square formation, 4-4-4-4, imagine that you are a skin filling with air and lifting just off the floor, as you breathe in and hold your breath. Then, as you breathe out, imagine that you are made of lead and that you are sinking into soft, warm sand.

Concentrating on this idea is very restful, so don't let it lull you to sleep. Don't jump up abruptly after your relaxation — come out of it gently.

LESSON 3

The theme of this lesson is awareness and concentration. This means noticing the sensations and movements of the body as you go through the postures, and asking yourself how they are brought about. And improving concentration means slowing down the stampede of thoughts rushing through the mind and centering it on just one. Each posture also progresses to the next stage of its development.

Limbering

To your repertoire of limbering exercises, you can add the Cat Stretch. Kneel on all fours with knees together and hands below the shoulders. As you breathe in, turn your head under, at the same time arching your back as high as you can. Think of an angry cat. As you breathe out, look up at the ceiling, allowing your back to sag in the middle.

A further option here is to straighten and raise alternate legs as high as possible and bring the knee to the forehead. Kneel on hands and right knee and raise the left leg high behind you, head up and back hollow. Then bend the left knee and swing it under the body to approach the lowered head.

The Tree (Vrikshasana)

This time you should concentrate on your back, shoulders and hips and the muscles needed to balance in this posture. This lesson also progresses the posture to the next stage.

Limbering

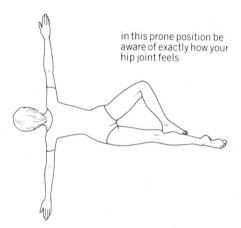

in this prone position be aware of exactly how your hip joint feels

Before you do the posture itself, limber with these two exercises.

First, lie supine, and take the hands straight back over your head, palms together. Stretch them, touching your ears with your arms and bring the thumbs into contact with the floor. Hold that position, flattening your back down, and close your eyes. Think how your shoulder joint feels now. It has to feel just like that when you are standing, balanced, in the Tree posture.

The second position involves concentrating on how the hip joint feels. Turn over and lie prone, take your arms out sideways, palms down, and stretch both legs straight back. Place the right sole on the inside of the left shin, pointing the knee to the side but keeping the body flat. Do this on the other side, too, closing your eyes and concentrating on the stretch in the hip and back. You are now ready to go on to the next stage of the Tree.

The posture

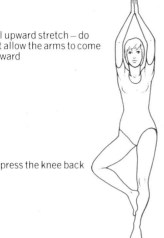

full upward stretch — do not allow the arms to come forward

press the knee back

Balance in the foot-on-foot position as before and take the hands into the High Mountain. Then move the top foot up on to the inside of the other shin. Point the knee out to the side and press it back — don't let it come forward. Try to lengthen the lumbar region of your spine as you do this. Make sure that the palms of your hands are flat against each other, not just touching at the finger-tips.

Keep your eyes fixed on a point and do not let them wander. Breathe in fully and out slowly. Hold the posture on each leg in turn for as long as you comfortably can.

If you lose balance, don't worry; just start again.

The Forward Bend (Padahastasana)

The Forward Bend here concentrates on stiffness of the lower back which many people feel after they have been sitting down, particularly in a soft easy chair which does not support the back or force you to sit up straight. While doing the Forward Bend this time, think about this part of your back and how any stiffness is caused. Between each vertebra and its neighbour there is a fibrous pad with a gelatinous core, known as an intervertebral disc, and each

51

time you slouch or slump in a chair, there is greater pressure on the front of this disc than on its rear. This may lead to a rupturing of the disc, when its soft core escapes between the vertebrae, developing the well-known slipped disc.

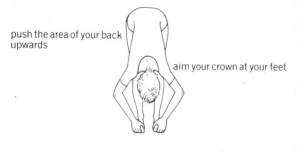

push the area of your back upwards

aim your crown at your feet

After bringing the trunk and arms to a position parallel with the floor and, with a second inhalation, lengthening both forward and backward, putting all the distance possible between the fingers and the buttocks, so that the legs slope slightly back, breathe out and let yourself drop so that you can grip your toes. Try then to lift the back of your pelvis upwards and to push the crown of your head onto your feet, gently bending your elbows.

The Stretched Triangle
(Utthita Trikonasana)

Again, it is the hip joints which have to be considered in this posture.

Limbering

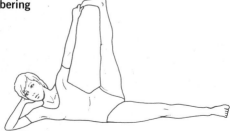

flatten your armpit to the floor — you will balance better

52

Before doing the Triangle itself, prepare for it with this posture, called Anantasana. Lie on your right side, both legs straight out and the head supported on the right hand. Push the elbow away so that your armpit touches the floor, as this gives better balance. Draw your left foot along the top surface of your right leg, touching it for as long as you can, until you can grip the toes with your left hand. Breathe in and straighten the leg, retaining your grasp and making sure the leg is quite vertical. This exercise frees the hip joint. Do this on both sides to prepare the hip joints for the Triangle.

The posture

Now do the Triangle as in Lesson 2, but concentrate on your hip joint and correct any tendency to turn the trunk during this posture or to lean forward. If you bend your foot correctly, in two pivoting movements as described in Lesson 1, you will feel movement in the socket of the hip. Don't look down at your foot and don't allow the trunk above the pelvic girdle to turn either.

Try finding the hip joint with your fingers and see if you can feel this internal rotation. Push the hip well out and feel the stretch as you reach out over the turned foot.

Now, instead of looking along the rising arm, look at the hand which is descending either to your ankle or the floor. Still keep your arms and shoulders at right angles to the floor and do not lean even slightly forward. Then look from the lower to the upper hand. Your neck will feel very taut. Breathe in and come up. This time look along the hand which is rising and watch it all the way as you bend to the opposite side. There should now be less tension in your neck.

As you bend over, notice the tension in your upper thigh muscle and knee-cap. Try to release it. Throughout both sides of the posture concentrate on holding arms and shoulders straight up from the floor. Do not come forward. It is easier but wrong, and this lesson is concentrating on correcting any faults as you think about the movements of your body during the posture. Let your breath flow steadily and count the number of times you breathe out. Make certain the number is the same when you repeat the posture on the opposite side. Inhale deeply and exhale long.

The Single Leg Forward Stretch
(Janu Shirsasana)

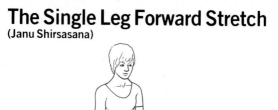

In this posture, too, the change in position from the last lesson is very slight, but nevertheless makes an important difference to the feel and effect. Whereas the sole of the foot pressed against the thigh in earlier exercises, now it is the ball of the foot. This makes the bent knee travel 4 or 5 cm backwards which extends the stretch much more than you might expect.

The toes are held so that the heel is free to move forward as the leg is lengthened. Rock the body slightly from side to side to allow it to lengthen, but don't let the ball of the foot creep under the thigh.

When in this posture, concentrate on keeping your back flat. As you stretch forward harden the muscles, both dorsal and abdominal, then, as you allow your trunk to hinge down to the leg, relax them. With each intake of breath flatten and lengthen, with each exhalation relax.

Next concentrate on the hip of the bent leg and, as you stretch, try each time to bring the knee down on to the floor. Finally, think about the hamstrings and the sinews being stretched in the underside of the straight leg.

Hold the posture for seven breaths on each side and you will find that you can gradually relax muscular tensions. Only then should you drop your head on to your knee.

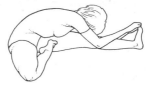

Sitting Rotation (Matsyendrasana)

the elbow presses against
the knee pushing it aside

This stage of the posture is called Ardha Matsyendrasana. 'Ardha' means half, so you are now well on the way to performing the complete Sitting Rotation. The purpose of this exercise is to stay erect whilst twisting round, freeing the hip and mobilizing the shoulder joint. To get the best results, make sure you sit firmly on both buttocks throughout and keep your shoulders level.

Sit with your legs in front of you. Draw up the right foot to the level of the left knee and then cross it over the knee. Holding the raised right knee, straighten your back. Turning slightly to the right, place your right hand behind you, close to the body with fingers pointing away from you. You will realise that you have twisted your body round the spine in three different areas. First, the lumbar region as you rotated at the waist, then as your hand was placed on the floor the shoulders, dorsal region, turned. Finally, as you turn the head to look back over the shoulder the cervical area is revolved.

Breathing in, take your left elbow across your right knee. Breathing out, push the knee aside and grip the straight leg just below the knee. Look back over your right shoulder. Try to keep the right foot and left leg parallel and close to one another. Rest and do the posture in reverse.

Concentrate on the movement of rotation. As you breathe out, press your elbow against your raised knee to help you twist further. Remain in the posture for seven to ten breaths, noting your own areas of tightness. They may be in the foot, the lower spine, the shoulder or the neck. Try to relax the areas that feel tight.

55

The Shoulder Stand (Sarvangasana)

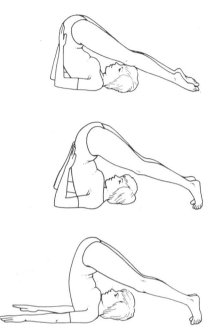

Here again the aim is to correct the posture as you have learnt it so far before proceeding to the full Shoulder Stand. Start with the Half Candle and go into the Plough, as before, the feet touching the floor behind your head, if they will, and your back still supported at the waist by your hands. Now do two things to correct this posture. Make sure that the soles of your feet are at right angles to the floor by pointing the toes away from your head, and bringing the heels back above them. This will bring your back erect and lock your chin more firmly against your chest. Then remove the hand support, taking the arms straight out on to the floor.

The breathing in this posture, particularly if you are overweight or heavily built, will be principally in the thorax, the rib-cage being moved consciously to its fullest practicable extent, and you may feel some restriction.

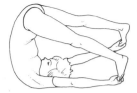

The following dynamic, called the Split Plough, should relieve the difficulty. It will also balance the weight on the shoulders better, so it is advisable for everyone to practise it. Swing the arms out and back to grip the toes with the fingers and, breathing in deeply, part the legs as widely as possible, holding on to the toes and keeping the legs and arms straight. Concentrate on your neck and shoulders and on balancing the weight immediately above them.

Even if you should have a tendency towards high blood-pressure, you may do these Plough postures providing, of course, that you do not strain by struggling to make your feet touch the floor before you are ready for this. If you find difficulty here simply let your feet hang in the air behind you as low as you are comfortably able to, though you may reach the hands back and pull them to the floor in the Split Plough. Treat this posture as a test to indicate whether you should or should not proceed into a fully inverted posture such as the complete Sarvangasana shown in the next lesson. If you can, with a minimum of discomfort, hold a Plough (Halasana) over a period of thirty gentle breaths you are ready to attempt the complete posture. If not, continue to practise the Plough and do not feel discouraged for this asana will do so much for you.

It will apply a toning pressure to the region of the thyroid and parathyroid glands giving them an essential supply of fresh blood. This in turn will affect your metabolism and the resulting improvement in your body's use of its food will regulate your weight. Its massaging action discourages the accumulation of abdominal fat, improves the whole digestive process and aids elimination of waste. Halasana is well recognised as a relieving agent for varicose veins, now understood to be caused by intestinal blockage, arthritic pain in shoulders and lumbago.

The Cobra with further dynamics
(Bhujangasana)

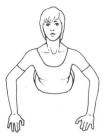

So that you become fully aware of the muscles which are used in this posture, they are now brought into play in turn. Start from the beginning of the posture, drawing the hands gradually in towards the head and finally taking up the full posture with hands under the shoulders. Hold this posture as long as you can without strain and then relax. Repeat the full posture, this time bending the knees and raising both feet up, the toes pointing upward, in the dynamic described in the last lesson. Again, don't try to hold the positon for too long.

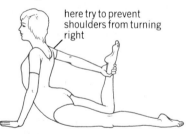

here try to prevent shoulders from turning right

Repeat the last dynamic, but this time bend up only the left leg, keeping the right one stretched straight out behind you. Reach back with the left hand to grasp the left ankle, supporting the posture with the right arm only. This is a very strong movement. If you find it too energetic, move your hands a little way forward and try again; remember that yoga is not designed to bolster your ego. Stay in this attitude long enough to note the tension in the spinal muscles of the lumbar region and the lower dorsals. Relax thoroughly in

the Swimmer position (see page 29) before repeating the
Cobra dynamic on the right side.
The upper dorsal muscles are also used in the Cobra. To
bring these noticeably into play, lie in the prone position,
hands at your sides, palms up. Raise the left foot and grasp
the ankle with your left hand, as before. Inhaling, lengthen
your neck and raise head and chest as high as possible.
Your shoulders will want to turn but do not let them. This is
where you use these muscles. Don't turn your head either.
The head and shoulders must face forward throughout.
Relax very thoroughly again before grasping the right ankle
and repeating this movement on the other side.

Breathing

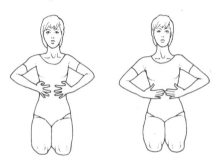

You can test your breathing and whether the movements of
your body are correct by placing your hands over your
abdomen or round the lower ribs, as illustrated. You can
also do this lying in the supine position. For abdominal
breathing, start with your hands over your abdomen, finger-
tips together. As you breathe in, the rib-cage should be kept
as still as possible and the abdominal region should expand
so that the fingertips part. As you breathe out, the abdominal region contracts and the fingers come together again.
This movement, which gives room for the large diaphragm
muscle to extend downward, is not just a pushing forward of
the stomach but an all-round expansion, including the
flanks.
In thoracic breathing, the hands are placed round the
rib-cage. The abdomen is flattened and kept flat, and the

hands can detect the extent of rise and fall in the rib-cage as the ribs open to allow the lungs to expand on an intake of breath.

Relaxation

Lie in the supine posture, stretching to your full length. Hold you breath for a few seconds, then let the breath sigh slowly out and the tension fade from your whole body. If there are any parts of your body that still feel taut, concentrate on relaxing them by tightening and then releasing the muscles.

Take care that you thoroughly relax the facial muscles. Screw up the eyes, wrinkle your nose, clench the jaw and grin, tightening even the scalp. Then let the whole face relax. Repeat this until you feel really sure that tension has departed from each feature. This is particularly important because the brain areas for most of your facial movements lie along the cortex of the frontal lobe and if they are tense the possibility is that the cortex will, as a whole, tend to be more active so that the mental quietude which is so essential to relaxation may be disturbed.

Breathe in the square formation again and slow your breathing to a gentle rhythm, keeping it mainly abdominal. Feel yourself rising and sinking with your breath as you did last week. The next stage is Body Rotation, a very restful form of concentration — so much so, in fact, that you may have to say to yourself, 'I must not sleep', for relaxation, to be enjoyed, must be conscious. The Body Rotation is performed by taking the mind rapidly from one area of the body to the next in a logical sequence.

Concentrate first on your right arm: the thumb, each finger, the palm, the wrist, the forearm, the elbow, the biceps, the shoulder joint. Then go to your left arm: the thumb, each finger, the palm, the wrist, the forearm, the elbow, the biceps, the shoulder joint. To your right side: the right armpit, right upper ribs, right floating ribs, the pelvis. Your left side: the left armpit, left upper ribs, left floating ribs, the left side of the pelvis. Your right leg: the right hip, the right thigh, the hamstrings, the right knee cap, the right calf, the right shin, the right ankle, the right heel, the right arches, the right big toe, second, third, fourth, little toe.

Your left leg: the left hip, the left thigh, the hamstrings, the left knee, the left calf, the left shin, ankle, heel, arches, left big toe, left little toe. Your back: the skull, neck, the right shoulder blade, the left shoulder blade, the twelve dorsal vertebrae, the five lumbar vertebrae, the sacrum, the coccyx. Your front: the scalp, the forehead, the right brow, the left brow, the right ear, the left ear, the right nostril, the left nostril, the right cheek, the left cheek, the upper lip, the lower lip, the chin, the throat, the collar bones, the breast bone. Your organs: the lungs, the liver, the heart, the stomach, the pancreas, the intestines, the spleen, the kidneys, the bladder, the colon. (If you don't know where these organs are, look them up in a book.)

Do not go to sleep!

Relax for several minutes.

Come out of this relaxation very quietly and try to carry it with you all day.

Perhaps you will relax better if you properly understand the importance of relaxation to your well-being. Activity, mental or physical, gives rise to sharp awareness in the cortical centres of the brain and this is passed directly to the hypothalamus at its centre which controls your adrenal glands. These glands are thus caused to infuse adrenalin into the bloodstream, in order to enhance the activity. This you may think to be a splendid arrangement, but it does have a draw-back, for adrenalin also inhibits the repair of body tissue and so impairs the body's powers of recuperation. Consequently, after activity we must relax so as to cause the flow of adrenalin to revert to its normal rate. It may well be due to the fact that they spend so much time training and so little in positive relaxation that many of our young football 'stars' find themselves impaired with strains and sprains, spending, it sometimes seems, more time on the masseur's table than on the field of play.

LESSON 4

We all have different physiques, levels of fitness, degrees of suppleness, supplies of fat. Since we don't come in stan- dardized bodies there is no reason why our performance of the various postures should be identical. Postures are for people, and no one should feel that he has to struggle into a posture down to the smallest detail if it doesn't suit him. So the theme of this lesson is 'adjusting to you'.

The aids suggested in this lesson should only be temporary until you have got used to the postures and are able to cope without aids. Don't let them become a habit. This also applies to any modifications to the postures you may need in the early stages. As you progress with yoga your joints and muscles will become more mobile, so you must reassess your dependence on such aids and adjustments from time to time, so that you benefit fully from each posture.

Limbering

This new limbering routine is the Standing Limber which is less time-consuming than the limbering routine described earlier.

It is important to do these four exercises smoothly, starting slowly, with the rhythm of your breathing, and to relax after each one, breathing quietly.

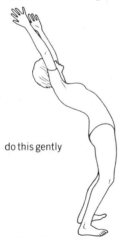

do this gently

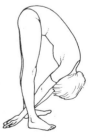

First, stand with the feet apart and bend backwards and forwards as in the first two pictures, touching the floor behind your feet on the forward bend. Then rotate the trunk right and left with arms at shoulder level and the head leading the movement. The third stage is like the Stretched Triangle limber, bending to each side. Finally, again with arms at shoulder level, bend to touch the left ankle with the right hand and then the right ankle with the left hand.

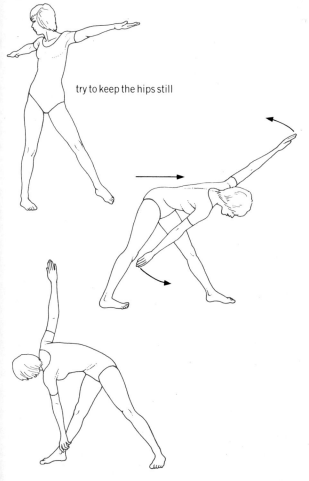

try to keep the hips still

Relaxation

The relaxation, too, is done standing. The straighter you stand, the better you can relax. Try standing with your back and heels touching the edge of an open door, and when you are satisfied that you really are erect, gently push the door away. Start to relax at the feet, balancing evenly between the ball of the foot and the heel. Brace and relax the knees, but do not bend them. Think of the space between your pelvis and rib-cage and attempt to keep this portion of your body in an upright line, its weight dropping into the pelvic 'basin'. If you have a tummy, you have a tummy; pulling it in won't make it go away. If your shoulders are rounded, pulling them back will not alter the fact. Such movements only set up tensions. Eventually the asanas will correct these faults. Look straight ahead and breathe quietly.

The Tree (Vrikshasana)

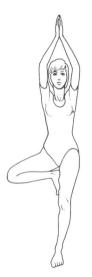

This time the full Tree posture can be attempted. You may find the balancing difficult, perhaps more so on one day than on another, depending on your state of mind at the time. If your degree of equilibrium leaves something to be desired at any particular practice, do not give up. Keep calm, and start again. You can, if necessary, steady yourself against a chair or wall in the early stages, and when you reach the final stage of the posture it sometimes helps to stand with your back lightly touching an open door. Then you can take several long, calming breaths and, when you feel really steady, take a hand back and gently push the door away. Then take up the full position again.

To go into the full Tree posture, start from the beginning with the foot-on-foot postures, progressing to the foot-on-shin posture, bringing the hands from Namasti to shoulder level, to Low Mountain and so to High Mountain. Take two breaths at each stage and finally bring the foot right up with the sole against the inner thigh as illustrated. Remember to keep the eyes fixed on one small object, the bent knee back and the palms together.

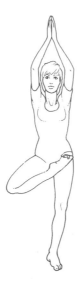

An alternative foot position is also shown here, the outer edge of the foot being fitted into the groin and the sole turned outward and kept in position by the backward pressure of the knee.

The Forward Bend (Padahastasana)

Limbering

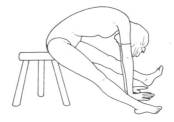

An alternative limber for this posture – indeed, it could be considered an alternative approach to the posture itself – is as follows. Sit, with your feet well spread, right on the edge of a low chair. Stretch up your arms and flatten your back, then, breathing out, hinge forward to lay your hands on the floor. Take several breaths in this position and feel the gentle stretch in your legs and over the lower back. Repeat this exercise, moving the feet gradually closer together.

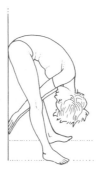

Next, stand with your back against a wall, the feet about 30 cm apart and 30 cm from the wall. Take the hands up again to touch the wall above your head, feeling the whole back flat against it, then, holding this straightness as you exhale, fold the trunk down to bring your hands onto the floor or to touch the wall as low as possible. This can be progressed by putting your feet closer together and closer to the wall.

The posture

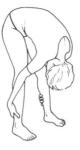

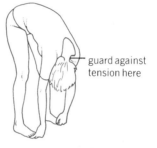

guard against
tension here

For the basic posture, place your feet close together and
inhale as you raise the arms overhead. As you breathe out
hinge the body at the hips, bringing arms, head and trunk
parallel to the floor. Breathe in again, stretching arms
forward and buttocks back. Look at your hands. Then
breathing out relax the body down to grip the toes. Direct
the base of your spine up and your head towards your feet.
Inhale deeply and exhale long, stretching gently downward. Keep your knees straight. There are modifications
which can be used if you have any difficulty with this
posture. The heavily built, thick-set person may find it
easier to have the feet parted a few centimetres. Or you can
grip your hands behind your ankles, shins or even knees if
you can't reach your toes. If you can reach your toes and
grasp them firmly by slightly bending your knees, this too
can be permitted — as you breathe out each time the legs
can be gently straightened.

67

The Stretched Triangle
(Utthita Trikonasana)

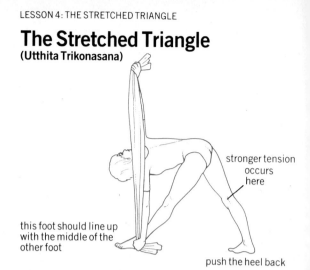

stronger tension
occurs
here

this foot should line up
with the middle of the
other foot

push the heel back

Start with the limbering exercise described in Lesson 1 and with the hip movement and sideways stretch shown in Lesson 2. Now refine the complete posture slightly by adjusting the position of the feet. As before, pivot on the heel and then pivot on the ball of the foot to turn the foot 90 degrees. Next, push the heel of the other foot back in the opposite direction so that the leg is tightened. Without allowing your body to come forward, try to put the palm of your hand on the floor as before.

A useful aid for testing the straightness of your back as you bend to the side is a scarf — or you can use a towel or a rope. When you raise your arms to shoulder level have the scarf gripped in both hands and passed over your shoulders behind you. Keep it taut and it will help to hold you back in a plane vertical to the floor. With this aid to hold you in position it is less important to look at the upper hand so if your neck still feels tense relax it by turning your head forward.

If you are practising these asanas with a friend you will find it beneficial to perform back to back. The arms are stretched sideways and intertwined so that your palms press against your partner's. Now when you bend to your right your companion will bend to the left, the feet being pointed accordingly

68

The Single Leg Forward Stretch
(Janu Shirsasana)

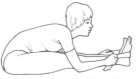

drop the elbows

This posture can give quite a lot of trouble in its fuller stages and once again a scarf, a towel, an old tie, or even a piece of rope can be helpful.

Hold the scarf in both hands leaving a certain amount of slack between them — you will be able to judge how much. As you breathe out, bend forward at the hip, looping the scarf over the feet and taking up as much of it as possible. Breathe in and stretch forward, rocking from side to side and holding on to the scarf as you push your head forward and elbows down.

If you are still finding it difficult to bring the bent knee to the floor, continue to do the limber recommended for this, and in the meantime you can put a small pad or cushion under the knee. But get rid of it as soon as you can.

try to lengthen the whole of your back

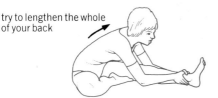

To do the full posture, you need to go flat on to your outstretched leg, with elbows bent to the floor. Begin as in earlier lessons, with one foot on the inside of the other thigh. Bend forward to grasp the ankle of the outstretched leg. Breathe in deeply and lengthen the whole body, rocking from side to side. Breathe out and let your abdomen go loose but continue to direct the crown of your head to your feet as you allow yourself to sink down on to the outstretched leg. With each intake of breath bend your elbows downwards and lengthen your stretch.

69

Sitting Rotation (Matsyendrasana)

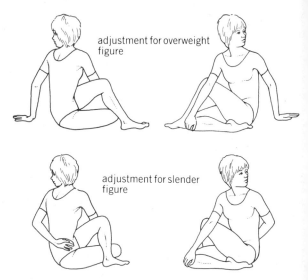

adjustment for overweight figure

adjustment for slender figure

Before you attempt the full Sitting Rotation, limber up by going through at least two of the earlier stages. Then sit with your legs straight out in front of you, in Dandasana. Take the right foot under the left knee and bring it up against your left buttock. Draw the left foot up and cross it over the right (bent) knee to place it flat on the floor. Breathing in, turn to the left, placing your left hand behind you on the floor, fingers pointing away from you. As you breathe out, take the right elbow outside the raised knee and straighten it to grip the right knee. With each exhalation press the right elbow against the left knee to aid rotation. Look over your left shoulder. Then repeat the posture in reverse.

If you are overweight, you can make an adjustment to the exercise. Still keeping the foot crossed over the knee which is bent on the floor, take it forward so as to leave you more room in which to rotate the trunk and to ease the movement of the elbow over and outside the knee.

There is another adjustment for the more slender figure. Keeping the body upright, remove the hand from the floor and place it behind the small of your back, palm outward.

The Shoulder Stand (Sarvangasana)

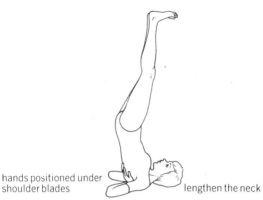

hands positioned under
shoulder blades
lengthen the neck

Many people find the full shoulder stand extremely uncomfortable because of the prominent seventh cervical vertebra mentioned earlier. Again, you can put a small pad under your shoulder or fold your mat to support and cushion this area, if you find this to be so.

If you have difficulty in raising the whole body really straight up, work against a wall as described earlier, getting yourself into the position by moving your feet up the wall, and raising your legs vertically when you are supporting your back with your hands.

To go into a Shoulder Stand, start with the Plough posture. Make sure that your back rises straight off the floor and your chin is tucked in tightly. Move your hands down from your waist to your shoulder blades. Hold your back in position as you now raise your legs straight up. Point your toes and stretch up as high as possible, still pressing with your hands and keeping your buttocks tucked in. If you find it difficult to raise your legs from the Plough position, don't strain — bend the knees first, pointing your toes upwards, and then extend the legs straight up. Once in position, relax your feet into a walking position.

It is extremely important to avoid this posture during menstruation. The blood shed at this time, being more acid, could be harmful if caused to flow back by doing an inverted posture.

The Cobra (Bhujangasana)

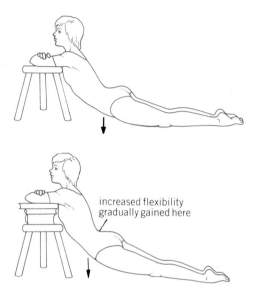

increased flexibility
gradually gained here

The performance of the Cobra will vary considerably from
one individual to another according to their proportions and
suppleness. It would be very foolish of a person with a waist
measurement of 36 inches and only some 5½ feet tall to
attempt to model his version of the posture on that of
another with a 26-inch waist and a height of some 6 feet. In
the case of the former it would be anticipated that the face
would tilt upward towards the ceiling only very slightly, if at
all. Nor would it be considered that his torso should rise
from the floor as vertically as that of the taller person, who
would also arch back the neck to gaze directly at the ceiling.
If you have trouble getting into the full posture shown in
Lesson 3, you can try this exercise to loosen your back first.
Find a small stool or hassock and kneel on the floor with
your arms folded on it. With your weight on your arms,
stretch your legs back and let your pelvis sag down on to the
floor. Do not hold this position for too long at first and bring
your hands to the floor one at a time before pushing back
into a Child posture. You can add a cushion, a book, then

two books as you become more supple, after which you will
be ready to go into the complete Cobra position.

Breathing

In this lesson the breathing practice consists of filling the
lungs, and alternate breathing.

To fill the lungs, first breathe out till you are really empty
and the abdomen is flat. Allow the abdomen to extend
slowly as you begin to suck in air. When you have reached
the limit of this movement begin the upward and outward
sweep of the ribs, filling the lungs, and finally take that tiny
amount extra by raising the shoulders slightly. Hold your
breath for about 3 seconds, then lower the shoulders, then
the rib-cage and finally flatten the abdomen again, keeping
it flat for another 2 or 3 seconds only.

Repeat this exercise for a few minutes. Remember,
though, that in breathing, as in any other aspect of yoga,
you should never strain. Decide for yourself how full is full.
Now repeat the exercise, but this time slowly raise your
arms from your sides as you breathe in through the three
stages, abdominal, thoracic and top-lobe. Raising your
arms above your head and placing the palms of your hands
together will lift the shoulders and slightly enlarge the
small top cavity of the lungs.

Our purpose here is that you should be fully aware of the
three sections of the lungs and the mechanism of breathing. After emphasising the sections separately in this
manner, continue your breathing using them simul-
taneously. Observe, too, that you are asked to 'extend' the
abdomen. This means sideways and even backwards, not
merely pushed out in front. That is simply the way to
develop a 'spare tyre'.

Alternate breathing is gentle, rhythmical and very restful.
Place the index and second fingers of your right hand on
your forehead just above the bridge of your nose. The idea is
to pivot the hand on these two fingers so that the thumb
descends onto, and stops, the right nostril, and then the
third and little fingers rock over onto, and stop, the left
nostril. That is the mechanics of it; now for the timing. Stop
the right nostril and inhale for a count of four through the
left. Stop the left and exhale for an eight-count. Do not

change: breathe in for four. Now change and breathe out for
eight — in for four.
Change nostrils: out for eight — in for four.
Change nostrils: out for eight, and so on.

Relaxation

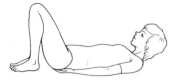

Take up the Corpse relaxation posture, Shavasana. Make
sure your shoulders are comfortably flat on the floor. If they
are not, take your arms further and further out from your
body and you will find that this takes the shoulders down.
When they feel really flat, keep your arms where they are.
Your back should also be firmly on the floor. If this proves
difficult, bring your hands over the back of your pelvis and
each time you breathe out draw in the abdomen and gently
ease the pelvic bone forward with your hands. You will find
that after several breaths the sacrum will fall firmly on the
floor and your back will be flatter. Remain with the knees up
like this until you feel set in the position. Then, very slowly
and gradually, ease first the right leg and then the left down
into the correct Corpse position, the feet dropping out
loosely. Return your arms to their best position for flat
shoulders.
If you find it uncomfortable to have your palms upward, as
some do, rest your hands on their edges. Some people feel
vulnerable in this open posture; if you do, cross your hands
on your chest. Feelings of vulnerability and relaxation do
not mix.
You should have made a slight double chin in order to bring
your neck and the base of your head as flat to the floor as
possible, but if this doesn't work, use a small pad under the
nape of your neck.

LESSON 5

Yoga brings harmonious unity of body, temperament and character, each at different levels, manifesting the vitality common to all life. This energy is universal. The yogi calls it 'prana' and Man absorbs it from food, sunlight, contact with earth, but mainly from the air he breathes. At its lowest level it vibrates in the activities of the body; at its highest, as intelligence. Capacity for prana is influenced by temperament and character. It is accumulated in serenity but dissipated by anxiety and anger.

The connection between respiration and emotion is well-known, so that in controlling prana (pranayama), we employ our conscious breathing. Accordingly, the theme of the final lesson in this book is breath control.

Begin your lesson with a short relaxation and as you do so become aware of your breathing. Set up a deliberate, gentle rhythm and imagine yourself in a transparent tunnel which runs the length of your body from head to feet. With each inhalation, picture a silvery wave of Pranic energy surging over and through you from the feet upward and as you exhale let this tide flow back from the head down. This will prepare you for two new forms of limbering which you may care to alternate with other backward and forward bends.

Limbering – The Swan

The Swan starts from the Child posture, the arms stretched forward as far as possible without coming off the heels. The hands should be placed a little more than shoulder-width apart. From this position, as you breathe in, bring your nose very close to the floor and take your head through between your hands, straightening your legs and coming up into a position resembling the Cobra except that the abdomen does not have to remain on the floor. With the tip of your nose you will then have roughly drawn the shape of a swan, starting at its tail, ending at its head and putting as much as possible 'in the water'. Now, as you exhale, starting at the head and coming straight down 'into the water', draw the bird in reverse, ending at its tail. You will then be back in the Child posture. Perform this limber three times, trying not to move your hands.

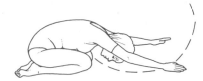

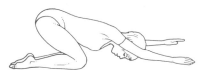

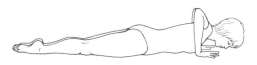

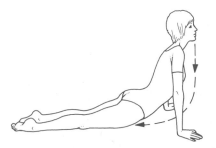

The Tree Posture (Vrikshasana)

Whatever dynamics you progress to in the Tree posture, and there are others besides the two mentioned here, never lose sight of the fact that this is a posture and not just a balancing feat. Maintain the upward stretch and increase your spinal length as much as you can. Always go into the posture gradually and never get annoyed or upset if you lose your balance. Your breathing will help your composure. In this posture it, too, should be kept in balance; it must be evenly divided between inhalation and exhalation and it must on no account become laboured. If the breath is calm, the mind is calm; if the mind is tranquil, the balance is good.

Count out a definite number of breaths — if you are in good balance, ten — and retain the posture for an equal number on the other leg.

Remember that the dynamics are for your good days. Otherwise stick to the basic posture which is much more important.

The dynamics

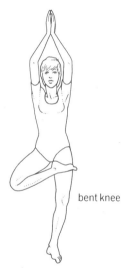

bent knee

The first dynamic concerns the raised foot, which is placed on the inner thigh in the basic posture. The raised foot should now be positioned, heel uppermost, against the groin as in the illustration above. The supporting knee may be bent, keeping the eyes riveted on a fixed point. If your ankle is stiff and the heel lifts as you do this, roll your mat up to support the raised heel and this will enable you, if your balance is good enough at the time, to bend the leg further. The other dynamic is the harder one. First achieve a steady balance in the position described for the first dynamic. Now close your eyes and try to visualize the spot you have been concentrating on.

The Forward Bend (Padahastasana)

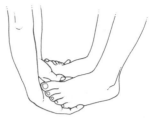

To go into the full Forward Bend, take the arms up with your in-breath, bring them halfway down with the out-breath and on the second inhalation really stretch, so that the hands reach forward and the straight legs slope slightly back. Keep your back as straight as you can but relax your abdomen as you breathe out, pushing your hands right under your feet. Bend your knees as little as possible. With each subsequent out-breath, bend your elbows and direct the crown of your head to your feet and the back of your pelvis to the ceiling.

This is a closed-circuit posture. As you breathe in, mentally direct the prana which you are gaining to the region of the solar plexus, which is traditionally regarded as its main storage area. Make your inhalation quite strong and your exhalation long.

During the exhalation direct the prana through the arms, up the legs and into that plexus centre. Before you breathe again, pause. It is during this brief pause that prana is generated from the breath. Stay in the posture now for ten or fifteen breaths, establishing that rhythm – strong, long, pause.

Everyone has his own rate and rhythm so do not try to match that of anyone else. Never strain your breathing. That is worse than straining your muscles. You should now be starting to relax in the posture whilst still correctly maintaining its shape. In the contraposture too, take prana to the plexus as you breathe out. Treat this control of breath and direction of prana very seriously. It is your longest stride forward so far.

The Stretched Triangle
(Utthita Trikonasana)

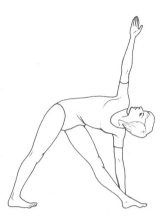

The final posture for the Stretched Triangle, pictured above, will require considerable practice. Look carefully at it and you will observe that both feet are now pointing in the same direction. To do this you start the posture standing with the feet together in Tadasana and take as long a stride forward as you are able to without lifting the back heel. Your feet are now in position but your body is not; it must be turned at right-angles to the feet. So, if you put your right foot forward, turn to the left. Now the arms can be raised, the hip let out, the right arm reached forward, the head turned and the posture achieved.

Doing the posture this way presents quite a problem, but the only answer to this is practice. Use the breath in this posture to help you relax into it, again establishing the rhythm of strong, long and pause. The strong breath is taken fairly quickly, the long exhalation is slow and the pause, to begin with, brief. As in earlier lessons, check whether any areas of the body feel tense while in the posture, but this time mentally direct the inflowing prana, with the long exhalation and pause, to the points of stress and try to hold the asana long enough for this to result in it becoming relaxed. Be sure to retain the posture equally on both sides and to bend to your worse side first.

The Single Leg Forward Stretch
(Janu Shirsasana)

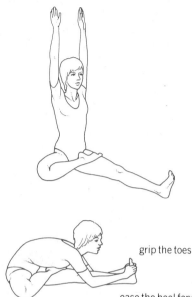

grip the toes

ease the heel forward

This is another closed-circuit posture. Again the breathing pattern in the retained posture is a short, strong intake; a long, slow sigh out; and a brief pause. The intake will be directed mentally straight to the solar plexus, and the prana will circulate, as you gently breathe out, along the arms and legs back to the plexus where it is held on the pause. Take seven to ten cycles of breath on each side. If you hold this posture for seven breaths you will probably find it becomes easier to maintain, as the body accepts the position.

The final posture of Janu Shirsasana shown on page 54 may now embrace one further feature. It will be noticed that, at last, the elbows have come onto the floor. If yours do not do so yet, do not strain to achieve this. As before, the ball of the foot only is placed against the inside of the other thigh, not the sole of the foot; the effect of this is to push the bent knee further back, lengthening the whole posture and further opening the hip joint. If this posture has been mastered, the foot of the bent leg may be placed, heel uppermost, on the groin of the straight leg, as shown here. This will increase the stretch and massage the abdominal organs more deeply. You should now be gripping the toes and pressing the outstretched heel forward, so extending the leg muscles slightly more.

Sitting Rotation (Matsyendrasana)

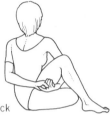

do not raise this buttock
or sit on the heel

When you turn your head to the right, put your right hand on the floor or behind your back, and twist to the right, the right lung has more room to function. So you should concentrate on taking air into this lung. The same applies when you do the posture to the left. Then the right lung will feel somewhat restricted, and so the breath should be consciously taken into the left lung.

You will notice most constriction and pressure in this posture in the vicinity of the navel and waist. Breathe in, filling the unrestricted lung; breathe steadily out, pressing against the raised knee to help your rotation; and pause before the next intake. During that pause, mentally direct prana to the tenser plexus area and concentrate on relaxing the whole of that part of the body as much as possible.

If you can now manage the full posture and are feeling supple, you can add some refinements.

You can rotate further if you take your arm over your raised knee and grasp the ankle of the raised leg instead of the other knee as before. This movement may be extended further by placing the fingers under the same foot. The very supple can pass the arm over the raised knee, bend it back under the knee and join the hands together, the other hand reaching round behind the small of the back.

81

The Shoulder Stand (Sarvangasana)

Because the body is upside down in this posture, the diaphragm is denied the support of gravity when it expands as you breathe in. You therefore have to consciously make it work rather than let it operate automatically as it does in ordinary respiration. When you breathe out during the Shoulder Stand both the ribs and the diaphragm are working against gravity, so you have to concentrate on working these.

Blood is taken to the cranium and face in the inverted postures, though not to the brain. But prana certainly is taken to the brain. As you inhale, mentally channel the pranic flow from the feet down into the spot in the middle of your forehead, known as the Third Eye, and hold it there in the pause before the next intake.

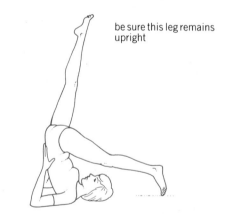

be sure this leg remains upright

When you are happy with your performance of the full Shoulder Stand, as described and illustrated on page 71, you can practise this dynamic.

Start in the Shoulder Stand as before, but keep your feet stretched high, rather than finishing by relaxing them into a walking position. Both legs must be kept quite straight at all times, and they are alternately lowered to touch the floor behind your head with the toes first of one foot, then of the other.

The Cobra (Bhujangasana)

You are now familiar with the Cobra posture and can turn your full attention to your breathing once you have worked your way into it. A good deal of the breath must be thoracic because the abdomen is kept in contact with the floor, which to some extent impedes the action of the diaphragm. Remember, too, that the dropping of the shoulders and stretching back of the neck right from its root encourages the filling of the top lobes of the lungs. Breathe evenly while performing the Cobra, with a distinct pause between the exhalation of one breath and the inhalation of the next. Think of prana being taken in with each breath from the soles of the feet up into the throat, and, on the out-breath and pause, permeating the heart and lungs and the dorsal spine. As you direct prana to these regions, think of relaxing them. The breath, and with it the build-up of prana, are the most important elements in the achievement of calm, controlled relaxation.

Breathing

knees as low as possible

In order to leave the thoracic cavity free to expand and contract unhindered, the spine must be erect. Apart from the Vajrasana position of sitting back on the heels, the cross-legged postures are best for maintaining the body comfortably upright while you practise breathing. The simplest of these is Sukhasana, the usual crossed-leg position where you sit with ankles drawn in close to the body and crossed. The only difficulty in Sukhasana, the Beginner's Pose, lies in keeping the knees as low as possible.

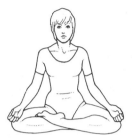

The Accomplished or Expert Posture (Siddhasana) is one of the best upright sitting positions and many say the most effective one for the practice of breathing exercises. Sit with your feet out in front of you in Dandasana. Bring the right foot up to the body, the toes pointed and the heel against the perineum. Place the left foot on top of the bent leg so that the outer edge of that foot fits into the niche formed between the thigh and the calf of the right leg. Similarly, you should find, the inner edge of the underneath foot fits the niche of the folded left leg. Try to keep the knees on the floor and lay the hands on them, palms upward. The back must be erect. Again this may be checked by taking up the posture against the edge of an open door, pushing the door away when you are satisfied that your back is really upright.

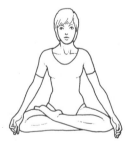

Many favour the Half Lotus Posture. If you choose this posture, be careful that, when you put both knees on the floor, you do not let the body lean and the spine warp laterally. The Half Lotus is similar to the Accomplished posture, except that the upper foot, instead of being fitted into the fold between the shin and thigh, is turned sole uppermost and laid on the thigh near to the groin. The hands can be placed as in Siddhasana or folded in the lap.

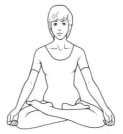

The ultimate posture is the Full Lotus (Padmasana). Starting with both legs stretched forward in Dandasana, pick up one foot, raise it high and put it down on the opposite thigh close to the groin, heel turned uppermost. This is then repeated with the other foot, taking this leg over the bent one to place the foot similarly on the opposite thigh. Notice that, in this posture, the knees are kept on the floor but are much closer together than in the other sitting postures given. The hands are placed on the knees in the same manner.

When you first achieve Padmasana do not attempt to hold it for a long period. Sit in it for a few seconds only and then release it. The length of time can be increased gradually as you become more accustomed to the position. To release the legs from this posture take each foot, separately, in both hands and gently slide it off the leg in front of the opposite knee so that circulation may resume normally. Remain in this position for a short time before stretching the legs gently forward and then, pivoting on the heels, rotate the toes above them in opposite directions in order to free the leg joints. This posture cannot be recommended for anyone who suffers from varicose veins or faulty circulation at the extremities.

Not everyone can achieve this classic asana. If you find it too difficult, don't force it as you could wrench a knee by doing so. Choose one of the other positions instead.

Practise whichever of these postures you choose both ways round equally. Change to another posture if it becomes uncomfortable.

Mudras

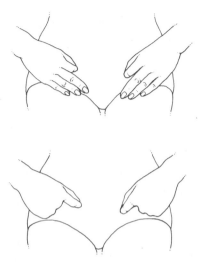

Mudras are a form of body-language which strongly influence the arousal of energy and the direction it may take. Not all mudras, alas, are yogic: consider for instance the shaken fist. When this mudra is performed emotion-based energy is directed into undesirable channels and begins to spill out with increased intensity. The great American psychologist, William James, insisted that action released energy, that towering rage occurred only after a blow had been aimed. Similarly the breathing function is increasingly energised by the simple actions of these mudras.

The three shown here are simple and effective. The first, Chin, shows points made by index fingers and thumbs, the remaining fingers extending rigidly forward. These points are pushed firmly into the mid-point of the groin. This point lies on the meridian relating to pulmonary action and the mudra encourages abdominal breathing. Chinmaya Mudra, shown in the second picture, is the same, and applied in the same way, but with the other fingers tucked into the palm. This stimulates thoracic breathing.

The third breathing mudra, Brahma Mudra, is to be used when the complete yoga breath is taken. The thumbs are

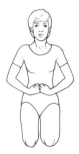

turned inward across the palms and the fingers wrapped lightly over them. The tip of each thumb rests against the bottom joint of the third finger. The lower joints of the first and second fingers should then be brought together, the thumbs pointing downward, and the fists so formed and touching should be located at the bottom of the breast bone, the elbows held against the sides. The breath should then be taken fully, starting with the abdominal, rising to thoracic and finally filling the top lobes of the lungs. Exhalation reverses this.

Relaxation

Relaxation will now have become deep and pleasant. Follow the same procedures that have already been outlined but now, before Body Rotation, perform what is sometimes known as Breath Concentration. This simply means regularizing the breathing into a light, unforced pattern and then, this established, beginning to use the count-down. Say to yourself, 'I breathe in – 26; I breathe out – 26. I breathe in – 25; I breathe out – 25 . . . I breathe in – two; I breathe out – two. I breathe in – one; I breathe out – one' and then take your awareness swiftly through a Body Rotation.

To finalise your relaxation it is pleasant and effective to allow the imagination to play around a restful situation. You may be rising and falling gently on a raft beneath a cloudless sky, quiet, peaceful and warm. But do not visualise yourself walking or swimming for such thoughts are the initiators of action and create tensions preparatory to it.

Benefits and Precautions

BENEFITS   PRECAUTIONS

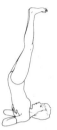

Shoulder Stands
Viparita Karani & Sarvangasana

Aids the circulation as gravity helps return of venous blood to the heart. Tones thyroid and parathyroid glands. Drains mucus from lungs into bronchial area for ejection. Gives relief to varicose veins. Rests abdominal organs from gravitation and increases their efficiency.

Best avoided by severe heart disease sufferers, people with hernia, detached retina, discharging ears. Not to be retained by those with high blood pressure. Inverted postures should be avoided during heavy menstruation.

Cobra
Bhujangasana

Improves chest expansion and encourages good breathing. Can be helpful for backaches and *may* aid the correction of spinal misplacement. Tones thyroid and adrenal glands. Strengthens wrists and neck.

Avoid after child-birth. Do not hold this posture if breath is short. Not for people with arthritis in hands or wrists.

BENEFITS   PRECAUTIONS

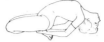

Fish Postures
Matsyasana
Gives stretch to all
leg muscles especially
in upper thighs and
knees. Supples spine in
dorsal area, opening the
chest. Hip joints are
freed and general
mobility of legs
improved.

If vertigo or a feeling of
sickness occurs
persistently, avoid this
posture.

Plough Posture
Halasana
Thyroid and parathyroid
glands are toned.
Stiffness in neck,
shoulders and lumbar
region is relieved.

If breathing becomes
laboured take feet from
the floor.

Supine Relaxation
Shavasana
Settles down the nervous
system. Helps to
reduce high blood
pressure.

Lotus Posture
Padmasana
Keeps hip joints free
and delays ageing.

Not for those with
varicose veins.

BENEFITS   PRECAUTIONS

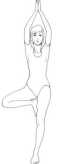

The Tree
Vrikshasana
Brings calmness of mind.
Strengthens the legs.
Improves carriage and
tones spinal muscles.

Support is advised for
people with weak ankles or for
vertigo sufferers. Should
not be done with knee damage.

Forward Bend
Padahastasana
Stretches the leg
muscles and those of the
lumbar spine. Massages
viscera and aids
elimination. Tones
adrenal glands.

Not to be done with slipped
disc. Backache sufferers
should do this very carefully
and without strain.

One Leg Forward Stretch
Janu Shirsasana
Good for prostate gland
ailment. Activates liver
and spleen. Aids
digestion and improves
appetite.

People with severe backache
should be careful not to
overstretch. Must not be
done with slipped disc.

BENEFITS   PRECAUTIONS

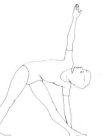

Stretched Triangle
Ut'hita Trikonasana
Good for loss of weight.
Massages flanks, opens
chest, increases
mobility in hip joint.

Should be learnt gradually.
Vertigo and knee troubles
will require gentle approach.

Kneeling or Child Posture
Vajrasana
A relaxing posture (Child),
and (Kneeling) a very good
erect posture for breathing
exercise. The Child posture
nourishes facial tissues.

Should not be held by
anyone with varicose veins.

Sitting Rotation
Matsyendrasana
Blood is taken to the
viscera which benefit from
massage. The adrenal
glands are toned. The
colon is stimulated.
Digestion and elimination
are encouraged. Shoulders
are suppled and relief is
given to stiffness and
aching here and in the back.

Should be avoided by any
person suffering from hiatus
hernia and stomach pains.

Glossary

Sanskrit Names

Asana: A posture which is held without strain.

Bhujangasana: The Cobra posture; literally the asana of the snake.

Dandasana: Sitting upright, legs stretched forward in L-shape.

Gorakshasana: Sitting between the heels.

Halasana: The asana which is shaped like a Plough, with feet taken over behind the head.

Janu Shirsasana: The Knee and Head posture. The body, from a sitting position, is taken forward along one leg.

Matsyasana: The Fish posture; the spine is arched up from spine.

Matsyendrasana: A sitting rotation. Refers to a number of postures which twist the trunk.

Mudra: A physical sign with mental significance to promote and direct energy.

    Brahma mudra: used in connection with full breathing.

    Chinmudra: connected with abdominal breathing.

    Chinmayamudra: connected with thoracic breathing.

Padahastasana: The forward bending posture in standing position.

Padmasana: A floor-sitting posture better known as the Lotus.

Prana: Universal energy.

Sarvangasana: The Shoulder Stand. Weight rests on neck and shoulders.

Siddhasana: A floor-sitting posture.

Sukhasana: A floor-sitting posture favoured by beginners.

Vajrasana: A posture which entails sitting back on the heels.

Viparita Karani: a half-shoulder stand (the Half Candle). The body is not straightened.

Vrikshasana: The Tree posture; a balancing exercise also.

Utthita Trikonasana: The Stretched Triangle posture; a strictly sideways bend.

Anatomical Terms
Cranium: The bones and tissues of the skull.
Cervical spine: The seven small vertebrae of the neck.
Colon: The large intestine.
Diaphragm: The great flat muscle stretching from lumbar vertebra to lower ribs and breast bone, forming a dome and moving in respiration.
Dorsal spine: The twelve large vertebrae of the back.
Lumbar spine: The five vertebrae in the small of the back.
Pelvis: Three bones which form the bone 'basin' at the root of the spine.
Perineum: Muscular area under the pelvis and just forward of the anus.
Sacrum: Five compacted vertebrae which fit into the back of the pelvic basin.
Thorax: Internal area bounded by the rib cage and diaphragm.
Venous blood: Blood in the veins returning to the heart.
Viscera: The organs, including intestines, contained in the trunk.

Index